CONQUER FOOT PAIN

CONQUER
Foot Pain

The Art of Eliminating Pain
So You Can Walk Through Life Again

JULIE RENAE SMITH, MPT

NEW YORK

LONDON • NASHVILLE • MELBOURNE • VANCOUVER

Conquer Foot Pain

The Art of Eliminating Pain So You Can Walk Through Life Again

Published in New York, New York, by Morgan James Publishing in partnership with Difference Press. Morgan James is a trademark of Morgan James, LLC.
www.MorganJamesPublishing.com

ISBN 9781642798463 paperback
ISBN 9781642798470 eBook
ISBN 9781642798487 audiobook
Library of Congress Control Number: 2019915185

Cover Design Concept:
Difference Press

Cover Design by:
Rachel Lopez
www.r2cdesign.com

Interior Design by:
Christopher Kirk
www.GFSstudio.com

Editor:
Cory Hott

Book Coaching:
The Author Incubator

Morgan James is a proud partner of Habitat for Humanity Peninsula and Greater Williamsburg. Partners in building since 2006.

Get involved today! Visit
MorganJamesPublishing.com/giving-back

To my family and friends:
you have been my change makers
and my obstacle removers.

Table of Contents

Foreword

As I was reading this book I was struck by the journey of the author and her ability to not only relate to the pain I have experienced but then take me on a on the path to relief. The body as a whole, broken into parts, and then rebuilt systematically can help anyone stop the automatic patterns that are keeping them from a pain free life. This book will teach you the steps you can take to begin assessing your body so that you too can be proactive in taking care of your health.

Chapter 7 is particularly important to pay attention to because it deals with your expectations, and how you manage patience when the pain is very much still present. Learning what the pain is telling you is critical in the process of easing anxiety that can come from not knowing what is going on or what to do to fix it.

Chapter 12 closes gaps and gives you a precise roadmap to begin living the life you want. It is a prescription for pain and if used in conjunction with all the other tools in the book and patience and determination you will have a body that begins working for you not against you. The case studies will help motivate you and help keep your faith in the times of slow change.

Julie masterfully weaves the stories of her pain, the journey she took to heal and the case studies that prove her results, with the remedies that will take your physical health to the next level... How would it feel to ask your body to accomplish something and know that it will work to do that thing? Run a marathon, compete in obstacle course races, playing tennis or simply getting out of your car and walking through the grocery store without pain. Use this book as a roadmap and a prescription for taking yourself not only out of foot pain but all of your pains.

Ari Gronich, "The Performance Therapist" Founder and CEO of Achieve Health USA LLC, is the creator and innovator of the Performance Therapy Academy Master Education System. Ari has been trained in disciplines within the fields of bodywork, kinesiology, nutrition, health, and sports therapy. He has over 25,000 hours of hands-on work and 5000 plus hours of education as well as having trained hundreds of therapists in the field.

Ari's passion is to inspire health professionals to shift the way they think so that they create a dream practice based on patient and client results. www.AchieveHealthUSA.com (321)541-0348

Ari Gronich
Founder and CEO of Achieve Health USA LLC

CHAPTER 1

Foot Pain, Ugh! Can You Relate?

Let's discuss your foot pain. This book will help you get to know what's going on and how it affects you. By understanding your foot pain, you can find the right solution, not a one-size-fits-all approach. How do you reconnect with your body instead of avoiding it? This connection will help you find a solution that works instead of going through just another cover-up operation.

CAN YOU RELATE?

- Do your feet wake you up at night if you have too much pressure on them or move just wrong? Lack of sleep can interfere with your concentration, how much energy you have, and your mood. Are you grumpy if you don't get enough sleep? I know I am.

- Do you feel like you hobble around like an old man for what seems like forever? All the while asking yourself, "Will it ever go away? What did I do?"

Often when people first get onto their feet after sleeping or sitting for a prolonged amount of time, they will hobble or limp until the pain settles down a little bit, but the pain may not totally go away.

- Do you feel like you are generally healthy? You possibly had a few minor broken bones as a kid, maybe some sprained ankles and pulled muscles over time, but nothing major and nothing that has lasted this long or been as debilitating as your foot pain.
- Do you find yourself saying, "I'm worried that this foot pain won't go away and I won't be able to continue doing all of the things I love to do?"
- Do you feel like normally you're pretty good at deducing problems, just not this time?
- You've tried insoles and specialty shoes, but they don't work—or at least not long term.
- You've tried resting for several days between workouts or runs, and just when you think it worked, the pain comes back.
- Have you googled how to solve this foot pain and tried everything recommended?
- You now own every foot massage tool known to man and every foot soak available—oh, and all of those ice and heat packs, too.

Temporary relief is the common theme here when you think about it.

- Do you find yourself saying, "Just when I think something is working and I can go back to running, I get only a few steps in and I have a hot poker in my foot again"?
- You have read several books and e-books about the causes of foot pain. Some of it you can relate to, but other things seem to have nothing to do with what is going on with your foot.
- Have you listened to several podcasts and researched all sorts of diagnoses for foot pain?
- Do you feel like sometimes they know exactly what you're going through—they have all the symptoms spot on—but then they talk about their solution and it's something you have already tried or something way off the wall?
- Meditating and manifesting a solution hasn't helped either.
- Have other people suggested that you do what they have done and "get the surgery" or injections?

That all sounds unnecessarily painful and gives you the creeps. I don't like the idea of having a needle near my foot, or a knife for that matter—do you?

- Are you willing to try just about anything?
- Would you like to find an alternative to all this but just don't know where else to look or what else to try?

I worked with a woman who was in the same boat, without many resources at her disposal.

I saw this homeless woman walking up and down the street where I had my first office. Every once in a while, she would come into the office and inquire about the price of a treatment, or just look around for a price list. This happened over the course of six months. At the end of that time, she came in and said that she would like to book a treatment. She had collected and saved enough money so that she could get her treatment. She was excited about it. All she talked about was how she had seen so many people looking like they were in pain or limping when they went into my office and came out happier and walking easier. It shocked me that she paid attention to my clients and made me a little worried.

She then told me about this horrendous foot pain that she developed over the past few years since she lost her house and was now walking more (on the streets). She indicated that her foot pain was at times preventing her from walking where she needed to go. She didn't go into too much detail of her past, meaning I didn't have much information regarding past injuries to go on, but I deduced that she probably didn't have to walk around much in her "before life." She and I discussed pain and how the pain was her body telling her something. We also discussed different types of pain and how she was classifying hers.

She shared some stories about various body aches she had and related each story to a type of pain that we discussed. It was interesting to see her actively making connections. She and I then discussed how the body parts are connected (the nose bone is connected to the toe bone). She was fascinated by my knowledge and how easy I made it for her to understand. We then discussed ways for her to be able to check in with her body and what the sensations she felt meant. I taught her some of the basic stabilization and postural activities and taught her how and when to use them. We worked together to realign her body and her feet and went through some soft tissue techniques. She was delighted with how her feet felt when she left. She tried to pay me, and I told her to go get herself a good meal instead. She was grateful.

I only saw her one time after that, about a week later. She came into my office to tell me how good her feet now felt and thanked me again. I never saw her again after that. I like to think her new feet and body took her to bigger and better things. These techniques and skills can be used by anyone—even you.

Experiencing foot pain can prevent you from being able to stand or walk (this is worse sometimes than others), interfere with your ability to travel or get you where you need to go, and interrupt exercise.

If you can't solve this problem, are you afraid you will have to live with this foot pain forever, that you won't be able to go to yoga, work out, or run? Are you worried that you won't be able to travel anymore when you already have lots of trips coming up and places you want to see?

Often people make lifestyle changes when dealing with pain. Have you already limited your activities without even knowing it? Have you found yourself having this conversation: "I haven't been to some of my workout classes or meet-ups in weeks because I'm too tired and my foot hurts?" What a pain!

Are you losing time that you don't have to spare your foot pain? Have you also been losing time trying to find a solution so you can get back to your normal routine? Dealing with foot pain, or any type of pain for that matter, can be exhausting and time-consuming. It can slow you down physically, interfere with your concentration, and result in some monetary adjustments because you're taking more rides or driving places when you would normally walk.

"I need to find a solution so I can get back to my life. I don't have time for this pain. I'm busy or at least try to be and it's taking me away from my work and I've not been able to make it to some of my meetings because I'm having trouble walking or I'm seeing yet another specialist." Does this sound like you?

If you could snap your fingers and change one thing, it would be to have your foot back to normal with no pain.

What would having your foot pain eliminated look like? You would be able to get back to your classes, workouts, and running. You would be able to get back in shape, stop feeling like a slug, try new classes and programs, easily make it to meetings, be excited about upcoming trips, and travel without worry.

GETTING TO KNOW YOUR SOLUTION

Learning what is actually causing the pain is important so that you can find a solution that works for you, not something that may or may not work for the "majority" of other people. One-size-fits-all solutions really fit no one. By learning to communicate with your body, you can find the cause of the problem. Using this practice, you can not only find the cause of the problem but also learn how to relieve it and prevent it from coming back. You can learn in just a few minutes a day what's causing your foot pain; how your body functions at its best; techniques that relieve pain; how to keep your body strong, stable, and pain-free; and how your brain can help you so that you don't have to go down this rabbit hole again.

Melissa came to me with significant foot pain that was preventing her from walking. She was given a diagnosis of plantar fasciitis by her primary physician (which, by the way, means irritation of the tissue on the bottom of the foot.) They basically told her that her foot was irritated but didn't really tell her why or what to do about it. She was told to stay off her feet and maybe ice them. We looked at what was happening. I helped her learn that a previous ankle injury and her knee injuries were all contributing to how she walked. We discussed how everything in her body was connected, from her feet to her head. Then we discussed the functional mechanics of the body; how all the parts work together. We discussed how she had some calf muscles that were trying to do someone else's job and how her hips were involved, too. Sometimes when we have a muscle that is weak or overactive, it is unable to complete the action it is supposed to do or tries to "help" with a different action. For example, if we have weakness in the innermost calf muscle (that is supposed to be helping us balance), then the outer calf muscle will try to help us balance and at the same time, try to extend the ankle. When these situations happen, we make unsuccessful movements or no movement at all.

We discussed and reframed how she classified her pain and different types of pain signals and changed her relationship with her foot. She was able to regain her body alignment, walk more efficiently, and use her feet in the correct way. By changing her relationship to pain and teaching her how to listen to what her body—specifically her foot—was telling her, she was able to relieve her chronic foot pain.

By learning how everything is connected, like Melissa, you will have the tools to eliminate your foot pain.

The body can seem like a complex system—foreign, as if it speaks a different language. With just a few techniques you can understand your own body. Your body wants to communicate with you; you were programmed to rush through your days so that you don't know how to listen to your body. You rush around so much and are in a zone of immediate gratification (you want everything yesterday) that you have more desire to escape than to ground. You disconnect your brain from the world. You try to find ways to distract yourself. You have lots of ways you do this: television, games, drinking, sleeping, and even your meditations take you up and out of your body and life (on a "vacation"). These distractions appear to help us slow our minds down and relax us; however, they actually interfere with how we live our lives. We become so disconnected from our bodies that we don't know what is actually happening in them. Most people are disconnected from the neck up.

CONSCIOUS AND UNCONSCIOUS MINDS

Our brains are seemingly our conscious minds, and, by contrast, our bodies are our unconscious minds. If we look at it this way, on the surface it makes sense that we feel like we need to be in our heads all the time, staying in the present moment.

This is actually counterintuitive, though. In order to be in the present moment, you need to be able to have both the conscious and the unconscious linked together. As you move through life, you store a number of things in your unconscious mind and your body by default. This begins when you are a kid. You fall down and are told to rub some dirt in it and walk it off.

Sometimes this works, but other times you are left with a small change to your body.

When you have emotional experiences, whether they are good or bad, you store these, too. That awesome adrenalin rush from zip-lining and the intense loss from the death of a grandparent—both are in there somewhere. That big deadline at work that's adding stress and the pressure to be at the school to support the kids are stored, too. You store this stuff in your unconscious because you "don't have time to deal with it all." Actually, you don't have time because more things are coming down the pipe. You disconnect from the experiences so that you can "get stuff done." You surge and plod forward taking care of all the daily tasks, the weekly tasks, the monthly tasks. You take care of the "most pressing" tasks, then tell yourself you will take care of the rest when those are done. The problem with this is that they are never done, and you don't take the time or make the time to address all of those things that you have stored in your unconscious mind/body. These things don't just go away; they make small, subtle changes in your body until all of the small changes have added up to a big one and it screams at you—like your foot saying, "Ouch! Don't step on me!" These small changes add up, and you don't even notice them. Learning to notice and to address these changes when they are small will help you avoid the big ones. It's important to reconnect with your unconscious and your body. This process works by helping you to do just that. It helps you understand what is happening in your body now and what happened in the past that is contributing to the current problem. By knowing what is truly happening you can find the right, effective solution for you.

FINDING A SOLUTION OR COVERING IT UP

Do you want to find a solution that's fast, easy, and not super time-consuming? The VITAL ME practice can help you to figure out what is causing the issue, give you actions to resolve the problem now, and tools to prevent a reoccurrence. Following each step-in order can give you some insights into what happened, why the pain hasn't gone away, and what to do next. The VITAL ME practice will take you step by step from your "vexing" pain to "experiencing" your body-mind connection.

Let's work together to figure out what is actually happening and get you back to pain-free and back to your normal life. Stop working through all of those solutions that "work for everyone." They are not really solutions at all; they are symptom cover-ups. Treating the symptoms does not fix the problem. You've seen this countless times when you take ibuprofen: it dulls the headache, but when it wears off, the headache comes right back. How about those ice packs? There is some pain at first, then the area is numb for a little while, and then when it warms back up— whoosh—the pain is back. This is what I mean when I say treating the symptoms. In order to get real relief that's long term, you need to find the cause of the problem—the true cause. Once you figure it out, you can treat that cause and prevent recurrence. You can stabilize, strengthen, and increase flexibility through your whole body because you no longer have anything interfering. You will also have the tools to be able to address the issue if it tries to come back when it is small so that it does not get to the screaming-at-you point again. Reconnecting your brain with your body will allow you to escape into your body instead of looking outside for relief. It will allow you to live in a stronger, healthier, and more stable body that is ready to conquer your world (or that new running program).

It takes only a few minutes a day to check in with your body, and it will tell you what you need to know every time. Let's figure out the cause so you can get back to your normal super-hero self.

Now you know how your foot pain affects you and you know that finding the right solution is possible. You also have a better idea of how you reconnect your body with your brain to help you find a solution.

CHAPTER 2

My Foot Pain Journey

L et me tell you a little about my journey and the bumps—big and small—along the way. I'm going to let you in on a couple of little secrets about me. I use this practice to resolve my own pain, and I have a superpower.

GROWING INTO MY SUPERPOWER

Little did I know when I was five that I developed a superpower. I was one of those kids who would give foot squeezes to anyone who would let me. Now, I say squeezes because they weren't quite a massage, but they still felt good. I found it fascinating that I could make people feel better just be touching their feet. I then progressed to taking my first formal bodywork classes when I was twelve. I took healing touch and reflexology (pressure points on the feet). I was hooked. I went on from there to study massage at the same time I was getting my bachelor's degree in kinesiology (the study of muscle movement and body mechanics). Sounds like I was on a track for success, right?

Well, life throws us obstacles, and we get only what we can handle. I was at college, away from home for the first time. Many things happened for me during this transition. This was an emotional time for me. I was happy to be responsible for myself and able to do what I wanted when I wanted. That was the great part. I also had some time where I felt lonely and confused. I sought some kind of companionship and even some guidance. I found this in my uncle. He and my aunt lived in the same city that I moved to for college. I was busy with my class schedule and I also worked, so I didn't have much free time, but when I did, I would go and spend time with them. I learned about essential oils from my aunt, which is knowledge I still use today.

I grew close to my uncle, and we learned a lot from each other. He lived life on his terms. He followed his heart and his passion in everything he did. He was a bodyworker, too. He was amazing when it came to combining massage and energy work. He flowed and floated through his treatments. I was the last person to experience one. When it was my turn to work on him that day, he relaxed into my treatment and gave me incredible feedback about increasing and decreasing pressure over certain areas, allowing me to improve my skills by working the tissue in a more effective way. He told me that it was my best massage yet. Shortly after that, having nothing to do with what I was doing, he had a stroke. He was still on my table as I finished up the treatment with the relaxing strokes at the end of a massage. I felt him go. His stroke was unexpected for all the people around him, but he may have known and may have chosen me to aid in his passing. This was a pivotal point in my career. I was not sure for quite a while after that if I could work on people. It felt like my calling, though, and I was good at it.

INJURIES INFLUENCING MY CALLING

At the same time that I was going through all of the emotions and grief around losing my uncle—especially in that way—I injured my knee. This was the second time I had significantly injured my knee. I went through rehab the first time, and I had been cleared to go back to my normal activities. In my first dance class after being cleared, and two days after I lost my uncle, I hurt my knee. I was keeping my movements small and trying to be careful, but it didn't work. I tore my medial meniscus and ACL—a scary diagnosis that I didn't fully understand. I investigated what exactly had happened to my knee. It seemed hopeless, and boy was it painful. I had to keep my leg in a straight brace for what seemed like forever (three weeks). As I learned to walk with the brace, I altered how far apart my steps were and the way I was stepping (one step was much bigger than the other), and since I wasn't able to bend one knee, I was swinging that leg way out to the side so I didn't catch my toe on the ground. I tried not to limp, but it's really hard not to when you have to keep one leg straight. Long story short, I had super bad foot pain on the other side. I had no motivation to do anything or even go to class because of my grief, and it was painful for me to walk or move. I was eighteen and wiped out.

It took me a little while to regain even a tiny bit of motivation, but when I did, I was off. I hung on to every bit of it. It started when I figured out what structures were affected in my knee. I poked around in my tissues, with my eyes closed, to see if I could feel what was happening where I was touching and if it was going anywhere else in my body. This was my first experience of really checking in with my body and learning to listen to what it was telling me. I believe as I was going through this process, my uncle was helping me and coaching me from the other side. I learned firsthand his energy work, happening through me. I changed what was happening in my body by listening to what my body needed. I rested when I had painful, tough days, and I stretched what was tight and strengthened what was weak. I learned to stabilize my knee so I could keep my steps even from side to side. I went through traditional rehab again, too, but that only served to frustrate me and teach me that they weren't doing what I needed. I designed most of my rehab program anyway, and they would just tell me to keep doing what I was doing. They did not change anything according to how I felt and tried to keep me in my brace for six weeks while prepping me for surgery. (That's how you fix a tear in an ACL or any other knee ligament—supporting the joint, right?)

I was out of my brace in three weeks and had more stability in my knee than was expected. My doctor and I discussed whether it was actually necessary to have knee surgery. At that point, unless you were a super sports star, they still filleted your whole leg open for surgery—not my idea of what was best for my body. The doctor said it would be better if we did surgery but that it wasn't strictly necessary. He warned me that the likelihood of me reinjuring my knee again was pretty high if we didn't "fix it." I decided that I was going to try to do without. You can always have surgery later, but you can't un-have it. In only a short time, I was back to dancing, running, and even weight training. I checked in with my body regularly and progressed slowly, but I was able to get my leg back to functioning and my foot pain on the other side resolved as I corrected my walking. The pain in my foot, as I found out, was not actually caused by my foot; it was just the part that took the load for all the other compensations I had made. This was not the end of my injuries, which, I came to understand, were all associated.

I was moving well and strong and stable. I was in my "new" normal, but I was not in my original normal. I was still working through some of the compensations I made when I hurt my knee. I slightly rotated my foot out to change the pressure on the inside of my knee. When I pushed during training, I needed optimal function. My optimal function was compromised, literally, so I was actually putting more pressure through my left foot than my right when running. I was also putting pressure not through the middle of my foot but more toward the outside, and the result was a fracture in one of the bones in the upper outside of my foot (the fourth metatarsal—see the foot anatomy picture here: https://bodyaffects.org/docs/Foot-Anatomy.pdf). I had made such gradual changes over time that I didn't even realize it until I started to listen to my body and what it was communicating with me. It was giving me signals of tension on one side of my leg and not the other, tightness in only certain areas of my foot, et cetera.

When I was beginning to walk again without a brace, I was walking on the very outside of the foot I fractured. Part of that was reacting to the pain still in my foot and part of that was in response to having worn the walking boot and how it changed my walking. Once that pattern started in my foot, the instability in my old knee pattern was exacerbated. My ankle became more and more jammed and my knee more and more unstable. My old pattern of knee injury was the same pattern just from the knee to the foot. They made each other worse. I wasn't even aware that I was still asking my knee to be unstable and my ankle to be stable. After the knee became a bigger problem, I learned to listen to my body. I remembered to check in with my body. I could feel my outside hamstring (the back of the thigh muscles) was tighter than my inside one. I could feel my quadriceps (the front of the thigh muscles) were not really contracting, being weak, so my knee stabilizers were not working. I then was able to feel what was wrong so I could make changes to the patterns decreasing my knee instability, letting my ankle become unstuck and allowing my foot to move in the normal heel strike to toe movement.

Then, when I was thirty-three and training for an aquathlon, something else happened. I was ready. I was in the best shape. I was going for a personal best. I was doing some last-minute speed drills and was going to start my taper the next week. My race was only two weeks away. My pool speed workout felt really good, and I felt strong when I got out. I went to the track, still in my swim skin so I could practice that transition, and I felt great completing my speed drills there, too. Even though I had felt great during the workouts, afterward my foot was hurting. It was achy when I did my other stretches and really sharp when I took too many steps in a row (about four). I thought I was doing everything right and felt good—where did this come from? I thought maybe my foot was tired and I just needed to stretch it out, maybe do some massage. Off I went to the rest of my day, sort of forgetting about my foot after I did a cool down stretch and self-massage. I forgot about my foot as I was treating my clients; however, every once in a while, I would step back and—wow!—a zinger would get me. It was a super sharp pain that seemed to go right to my brain.

After a couple of days of that—with the "zingers" getting more frequent and worse—I got my foot looked at. I wasn't training either. I didn't feel like I could or that it was a good idea. This was an issue. The doctor took an X-ray. She then strolled in, saying that she didn't see anything on the X-ray and that I should just rest and stay off it. I replied that I was in training for a race and needed to stay on track and that I was on my feet all day for work. She simply shrugged her shoulders and said if I rested and stayed off it, it would be fine. I left there wondering whether she was right, and I just needed to rest or if something more was happening.

I work with injuries all the time, and the whole situation seemed strange. I walked back into the office and asked if I could see the X-ray. I knew where the pain was and how to read an X-ray. They finally let me see the X-ray about thirty minutes later. I thought, "It's my X-ray. I should be able to see it, and I should've been given a copy anyway." As I looked at the X-ray, I could see that there was a small fracture in one of my foot bones. The doctor had missed it. I asked to see the doctor again, which was like pulling teeth. She finally came in, and I pointed out the fracture and asked what she thought now. She stuck with her original statement of not seeing anything and that I should just stay off it for a while. I left furious. I not only was able to see the problem, but I was also dismissed. This was not going to work. I then followed up with a doctor friend of mine who prescribed a walking boot for me. Needless to say, I was not able to keep up my training and did not get to compete. I was devastated. After all the work I put into my training, I was confused about how the injury actually happened. I had felt good and strong during my workouts.

My foot healed in about six weeks, and I went back to a lighter training routine with more swimming than running. After a little while, I noticed that my foot still wasn't right and some of the pain was starting to come back. But I knew there was no way I had refractured it.

Round and round I went with my foot pain. I did research and really paid attention to how I moved. I had a previous set of injuries that I had written off as recovered. I was a kid when they happened and had seemingly recovered from them. But that was not the case.

I had to make some behavior changes. I got out of my workout routine. I had to walk in a boot, so I made walking changes, too. These were the little changes that occurred first. As I got back into my routine and out of the boot, I also made some bigger changes. I convinced myself that my foot was going to take a long time to heal. I thought my movement patterns were good before this happened, and when it happened, I noticed my movement patterns weren't great, so I convinced myself that I was not in very good shape and that I didn't know what I was doing so maybe I shouldn't compete in an aquathlon. I have not actually competed again. As I worked through this part of my own ability to pay attention to my body's communication, I noticed that these major thoughts and emotions really did change my behavior and how I worked out, what I chose to do, and how often I did things. There were several years where I didn't compete because of these thoughts and emotions, and I didn't even realize it. I could have competed. I've actually been in better shape than I was when my foot injury happened many times since then.

As I adjusted my interpretation of my pain in my foot, checked in, and paid attention to what my body was telling me, I decreased my pain levels pretty quickly, so what I experienced was productive discomfort (pain signals telling me I was making good changes instead of telling me to stop the movement) and soreness (muscle fatigue) instead. As I checked in, I identified what patterns I was running. One of my main patterns was a rotation of my left shin bone (tibia) to the outside. When running that pattern, I was walking on the outside of my left foot, which put pressure on the outside of my left knee. This also led to increased muscle tension and ligament distress on the inside of my left knee and few more, well a lot more other things up the chain. I was also running the stable ankle, mobile knee and mobile opposite knee program, which interfered with my exercise and my foot function.

As I applied some stretches and some stabilization exercises, I decreased and stopped those programs. As I had more and more success in relieving the foot discomfort and stabilizing the knee, I returned to my activities more quickly than I thought was possible, and it created a snowball effect; the more success I had, the more success I had.

I did run into a little bit of "I feel better" amnesia, too, which is how I know it exists, and had some setbacks. During those brief setbacks, I refocused on checking in and really listening to what my body was telling me, relearning to experience my body and what it was communicating during rest and activity. It's important to be able to check in with your body and what it's experiencing, no matter what activity you're doing, not just when you're sitting still. The more you change your pain interpretations (your classifications of pain), learn to communicate with your body (your right brain), and tell your left brain what to do, the faster you will be able to heal and the better able you will be to seamlessly make adjustments to live in your optimal function.

I regularly check in with my body and complete the stability activities I need to return to my favorite activities. I continue to work through this practice. It allows me to live relatively pain-free most of the time. I, like most people, continue to do crazy or stupid things, so I rely on my ability to check in with my body when something comes up in order to reprogram my body and get back to my optimal functioning. That is why I call it the VITAL ME practice. These tools will allow you to continually work with your body because you continue to move and do new things. We don't live in a bubble. My body-mind communication is crucial. I am now much more aware of when my body tells me something is not perfect, so I can correct it right away. You will continually need to make changes and reprogram your body.

We'll discuss the patterns I'm talking about later in this book. I recommend coming back to my story after we discuss a new pattern or tool, as it will help you relate to your own story and how to put these tools into use.

MY JOURNEY, CONTINUED

I continued on my bodywork journey first by working on my own knee and compensatory patterns and then by continuing to study and work in massage therapy. This treatment of my knee really inspired me to go in the medical or rehabilitation direction with my bodywork. I learned to combine the few modalities I knew to optimize the benefits. (Massage, reflexology, foot joint mobilization, and the ability to use energy work—like my uncle—and body check-ins.) I continued on the pathway of my calling despite of and because of the challenges that I faced.

A few years after all that, I graduated with my kinesiological sciences degree, specializing in biomechanics and neurological reprogramming. (That means I know how the body is supposed to work in an optimal way.) I worked in my practice to help people with body stabilization and optimization through kinesiology, soft tissue manipulation, and energy work. I have since added multiple massage modalities from around the world, fascial and myofascial techniques, posture connections work, alignment techniques, and a physiotherapy master's degree from England. All this means is that I know how to do a lot of weird, cool stuff.

WHY CHOOSE ME TO HELP YOU?

For you, though, it means that I have the knowledge and superpower to show you how to feel like you're in your sixteen-year-old body, back when nothing hurt, and everything worked. It starts by learning how to communicate with your body.

I've taken myself through several injuries since then. Moving through regular check-ins with my body, learning new ways to communicate with and listen to what my body is telling me to re-stabilize my body. I experienced periods of pain that I needed to attend to. I'm not telling you that I magically made it, so I don't have pain; I have just figured out what to do about it when it's small and easy to fix instead of waiting until I have a big problem. I check in with my body daily or multiple times a day, depending on what is going on. If I don't stay in touch with my body and stay mindful of my alignment and stability, stuff hurts. I have "I feel better" amnesia and forget sometimes, but I'm active and sometimes do stupid things, so my body will remind me if I'm not paying attention with a little nudge of pain. I have some periods where I do my postural and stabilizations activities every day. This allows me to run and swim and do what I want when I want with my body. I have other periods when I need to do my exercises or stretches more than once a day and still other periods when I can do them once a week.

Have you ever had "I feel better" amnesia? Have you ever had pain you just ignored, hoping that if you forgot about it, it would go away? Me too. Sometimes these avoidance techniques work, right? No, not really. These things have a way of sneaking up on us and getting in the way all over again. It's best to address things as they come up; whether it's physical or emotional (yes, it's okay to have emotional injuries), they will come back if we store them.

I have been able to pass my knowledge on to others as well. Now, I want to help you.

I have helped countless people with the VITAL ME practice and in my therapy clinic learn how to check in with their bodies and learn to listen to what it's communicating. I have helped people learn how to look at what is happening and what happened in the past that may be contributing. And I have helped people learn simple tools they can use daily, in only a few minutes, to keep their bodies strong and stable.

I love what I do, and I want to help as many people as I can. Using body check-ins and knowing how everything is connected, we can figure out what your body is telling you, how to re-stabilize it, and how to get you back to your best body. And you can do this as a practice, continually correcting and reprogramming as you learn new things, experience different issues, do stupid things, and live your life. You won't necessarily be able to be pain-free all the time, but you sure can be most of the time. Remember, pain is the body trying to tell you something, so listen! If you don't know how, you can learn just like I did. Hopefully I can shorten your journey so you can learn this practice and these tools in just a few chapters instead of more than twenty years of stumbling around, learning more techniques, sustaining injuries, and figuring out how to solve the puzzle or set the dominos back up, as the case may be.

Now that you know more about my secrets, my pain, and my superpower, I would be honored if you would allow me to help you on your journey to conquer your foot pain.

CHAPTER 3

The Tool Belt.
What Do I Need to Know to
Relieve My Foot Pain?

I would like to give you a little taste of my VITAL ME practice; this is the practice I use to correct my pain and movement problems. I use this practice every day, and I would like to share with you how it works. You will move through various steps that will help you understand what is causing your pain and what, from your past, may be contributing to what is currently happening. Then you will get an idea of what a pain-free body looks like and how you compare. Next, you will get an idea of how to change your interpretation of pain, how to address your pain, and techniques that will help you now and in the future. All these steps will help you obtain and maintain your best body and keep your mind connected too.

HOW TO GET STARTED

Resolving foot pain to get back to normal, exercising, sports, travel, et cetera, is crucial. By using the VITAL ME practice, you will have some tools to figure out what is actually contributing to and causing your pain. This is called a practice because you will find that you will go back to and move through these steps multiple times. As you move through the steps, you will find you become better at the practice and will be able to move through the steps more quickly and more effectively.

It's important that you move through the steps in the order that I have laid out. It's difficult to know what exercises to use if you do not first understand what is going on. Knowing where you are starting out is crucial. Then knowing what past issues or injuries could be exacerbating or contributing to the current situation or issue becomes very useful. Once you understand where you are and what other things may be involved, all of those things can aid your ability to check in with your body; they help you know where to look for information from your body. The more you know about your current situation, the easier it will be for your body to communicate with you.

I learned how important it is to communicate with my body as I was going through my challenges with my knee and all of the other emotions I had floating around about my uncle. I've also had several other injuries and issues since then too, and I'm glad I learned that lesson early. Communicating with my body has been a saving grace, or I would probably be half a bionic person by now.

THE VITAL ME PRACTICE STEPS

Step One: "V" — Vexing Pain

This step is about identifying your "vexing" pain; this is any pain that is frustrating, annoying, or worrying you.

- Is your pain stopping you?
- What is it stopping you from doing? Why?
- Is the pain only in your foot or is another area involved?

Often the problem is not where the pain is. Getting to know your pain is important, too. Knowing the type and severity of your pain can help identify what type of tissue is involved and how much of the body has compensated for the pain and/or injury. Knowing how you classify your pain and that you can change those classifications can change your experience of it.

Did you stub your toe on Monday and are walking like Quasimodo by Friday, but man, you're determined to not take any breaks? We often do things like this. Has anyone ever asked you why you're limping? And you say, "What are you talking about? I'm not limping. I've always walked like this." Then you start noticing that you are, in fact, limping and didn't realize it. You're in good company; I, too, have had this happen. In fact, this happened quite a bit after I hurt my knee the first time and after I fractured my foot. I know better, and I still do this.

Then, you identify any past pain, injuries, or compensations that could be contributing to the current problem. Sometimes old injuries rear their heads. Often as kids and young adults, we don't get injuries treated or even looked at. Sometimes injuries heal and don't need treatment and are truly healed and will never again be a problem. Very frequently, though, injuries only partially heal because we have done more damage than we thought and create compensations because of it. There are some cases where the original injury will heal, but the compensatory movements or strategies remain and cause their own issues that come back later. Sometimes the compensatory strategies we devise are complex, and we can get to a point where we think those compensation movements are normal movements; then they become the new normal. Sometimes the whole injury appears to be healed until we do something similar again. Then the whole mess comes back, and the new injury can be even worse because of the old one. Identifying these potential saboteurs can be helpful to really figure out the true cause of your pain.

Remember that old ankle sprain (or five, in some cases)? Sometimes those suckers come back to haunt you. How about that one time you fell off your bike, and everything was sore for way longer than it usually was? This means you did more damage than you thought. How about that time when you were showing off with some friends and ran faster and farther than you had in ten years? Yeah, the next day sucked pretty bad (but you didn't tell anyone—kept the ego intact). Your secret is safe with me. I've been known to do some stupid things in the name of showing off, too. These things can come back to contribute to some "new" pain or pain that seems to come from out of nowhere.

Mary had a major dance injury; she had a sprained ankle on one side and a very painful bone spur on the other. She went through all sorts of dance-specific physical therapies. She was icing after every dance or walking too far and was eating ibuprofen like it was candy. We were able to restructure her alignment with body-mind education, soft tissue work, and joint manipulation. We worked through her strain with scar tissue realignment so she could stabilize her ankle again, which changed the amount of pressure that she put through her other foot and toes, in particular. She was able to incorporate stability exercises into her routine at home. She learned how everything was connected and learned how to actually listen to what her body was communicating instead of just working through the pain as she had previously been taught. I taught her a good compensatory pattern that allowed her to accommodate for her bone spur so that she could continue dancing in a pain-free way. As she stabilized and checked in with her body, she reabsorbed her bone spur because her body no longer felt like it had to protect that toe. She also learned to reclassify her pain signals, so she knows when she has an injury or tissues at risk and when something was just overworked.

It's important to address all of the contributing factors, such as ankle sprains—new or old—so you, too, can become pain-free.

Step Two: "I"—Improper Alignments

This step is about identifying any improper alignments you may have. When your body is out of optimal alignment, you know you have compensatory strategies at play. Knowing or learning what parts and how they are out of alignment can help you determine what is needed to remedy the issue. What is improper alignment, you ask? The body has a particular way it is put together. We do this in-vitro with our DNA strands. Our bodies and our brains know how everything fits together so it works. Sometimes imperfect movement patterns develop during this growth period. These patterns can be worked with.

Our head belongs in the middle of our shoulders and shoulders above hips. Our spine in the middle has curves of its own, which protect and facilitate the functioning of the nerves. Shoulders are even from side to side, down to elbows and wrists that move in the directions they are designed. The hips are even below the shoulders, and the knees and ankles stack on top of each other. The feet are glued to the bottom—and presto, a functioning body. The nose bone is connected to the toe bone. When body parts are connected in a funny way, like the shoulders being rotated forward (this happens when we sit at our desks too long) or the feet turned out to the side, you know you have a misalignment or improper alignment. These very often lead to discomfort and pain, as well as poor, ineffective movement patterns.

Did you know that if you lead with your head, you get there faster? Not really, but this posture is common and can create a ton of improper alignments. How about sitting with your legs crossed in a meeting, not paying attention, and now you've been sitting like that for thirty minutes. Getting up can be fun. That hip now feels like its glued on wrong and your foot's asleep, so it hurts to step down. Yikes! What have I done? We all do things like this, often several times a day (at least in my case). Knowing that you're doing this or going to do these things can help you prepare for them and make your recovery from "stupid" much faster.

Step Three: "T" — True Alignment

This step is where you learn what true (optimal) alignment looks like. Once you have an idea of what your body is supposed to be doing and how it should be linked together, you then can compare what it is actually doing to what it could optimally be doing. This will help you further identify what tenacious (stubborn) patterns you are functioning with that are getting in your way. You know the old adage "old habits die hard"? Well this can be true of old movement patterns. Sometimes, as I said, you are functioning with compensatory patterns without even knowing it because you convinced yourself that that's the "new" normal. Once you understand these patterns and true optimal movement patterns, you can begin to create a plan to transform one into the other. Preferably going from suboptimal to optimal and not the other way around.

Have you ever watched a little kid? They have beautiful posture with no effort. And they can run like the wind. Can't keep up with those little guys? That's optimal function at its best. Jealous? I know I am.

Step Four: "A" — Allow for Change

This step teaches how to allow for changes to happen so that you don't keep running those suboptimal movement patterns. One of the main ways you can allow for change is to check in with your body, that way you think the change is your left brain's idea, so it (your analytical judgmental brain) will get out of your way. Or you can tell your left brain how to interpret what is happening and still get it out of your way. It's only trying to protect you, usually from yourself. This protection often gets in the way when you try to reprogram. Your survival mechanisms catastrophize change and run the worst-case scenarios; so that part of your brain thinks you need to be in pain, say mean things to yourself, and have at least one failure a day to survive. This is not actually the case, but it's the worst case and you've survived that before, so that means that's how you survive. Why change it if you survived? Your brain comes up with some crazy things. However, if you can get that part of your brain out of your way, you can make meaningful changes to decrease pain and optimize movement patterns with the other part of your brain (the right brain) that's not trying to survive, but is trying to move optimally. When you check in with your body and right brain, you get the best information on what needs to be done to go back to optimal movement patterns and decrease pain by doing so.

It's also important to manage your expectations because unmet expectations lead to unnecessary failures and fights. If you check in with your body, it can communicate with you in a very real way and you can create expectations that are relevant and proper at the moment, hour, day, et cetera. This prevents unrealistic and unmet expectations. Change is inevitable. It's the only thing you can truly count on. Ah, entropy.

Have you ever noticed when you decide to do something, just intend to do it, and get started right away, everything seems to magically work out? Then, when you're trying really hard to make something happen, making all the plans, visualizing the end, and setting goals, but not starting anything, it just doesn't work, or you can't seem to get to it or get it done? When you resist or "try" to do something instead of just doing it, you convince yourself of all kinds of stuff, make all kinds of excuses, and get in your own way. When you just let something happen or change, it does, and you get out of your own way. This is why it's important to allow for change to happen. Communicating with your body can help with this and can take your left brain out of the picture.

Step Five: "L"—Learn Techniques

This step is where you learn some techniques to relieve pain, reframe pain, create changes in suboptimal patterns, reprogram patterns, and create optimal movement patterns that lead to feeling like you are in a younger, more functional version of your body. These techniques can be used when you have an issue all the way to becoming part of a daily maintenance routine. These exercises and activities seem small and insignificant, but if you incorporate them, you will feel like a superhero.

Steve has been practicing the VITAL ME practice for a few years now. He's in his late fifties and went snowshoeing with his thirty-something-year-old daughter and her friends. They couldn't keep up with him, and he was the only one not sore as heck the next day. He seamlessly adapted to the situation and has continued to work with the stability and postural activities that he learned so that he can move with grace. Superhero stuff. This practice will enable you to be the superhero in the group, like Steve.

Step Six: "M"—My Best Body

This step is about using these techniques to live in "my best body." They will help you stay there and make seamless changes if something small comes up. They will also help you figure out what is happening and what is contributing if something big happens. You will use these steps as a practice going through them as you need them. You will have the tools you need to be in control of your body and how you deal with, recover from, and prevent pain. Ever seen a toddler learning to walk? They look drunk. They wobble all over the place. Then, they finally get it and they're off and running everywhere! What they're doing is learning optimal movement patterns, reprogramming suboptimal programs and doing so with pretty effortless change. You can do this, too, not just with walking and running, but also with all the other activities you want to do.

Step Seven: "E" —Experience Body-Mind Awareness

This step is where you will experience body-mind awareness by learning the practice of checking in with your right brain and body so that you will spend more time functioning in optimal movement patterns and making seamless changes to stay there. Knowing how the body-brain connection works and learning more in-depth ways to cultivate it over time. The more you check in with your body, the more you will check in with your body, making it a habit (the good kind). This can eventually result in knowing what is happening with your body in real time so that you can be body-mind connected during all of your activities, with very little effort (it sort of becomes automatic). I've used this check-in method to be able to function doing all of the activities I want to do, to stay active, and to keep up with my crazy-fit dad while running, and all without having an ACL in my knee after more than twenty years. If I didn't know what was going on with my knee, I would have significantly more pain, I'm sure, and I probably wouldn't be as active as I am (and maybe would have gone down the surgery route, too). Checking in with your body can make a big difference (and it's pretty cool to communicate with your body).

The VITAL ME practice is a tool belt you can continually use to stay active, strong, stable, and pain-free. And to keep your brain on the same page as you are.

By using this practice every day, you can conquer your foot pain and get back to normal. This is a practice and an art that takes some time to implement, and it will get you back to your favorite exercises. The steps help you truly understand what is causing your pain and what else may be contributing. This practice will help you find your best solution to what is currently happening, give you tools to address any future issues, and help you stay pain-free.

CHAPTER 4

Vexing Pain— Why Do My Feet Hurt?

L et's discuss the true cause of your foot pain and why it hasn't gone away. In this section, you will learn how to give yourself a basic assessment, so you know what is going on in your body. (It sounds harder than it actually is.) With the information from your assessment, you will gain a better idea of what your body is telling you, what kind of pain you have, what that pain means, and why you should listen to your body.

PRESENT PAIN

Let's get to know your pain…
* Can you describe it?

- What does it feel like?
- Is it poky or sharp?
- Is it dull and achy?
- Is it numb and tingly?
- Is it hot or cold?
- Is it some combination of all of those?

Really take note of how it feels.

- When is it the worst?
- In the morning or in the evening?
- After you've been sitting for a long time?
- After walking or standing?
- Is it stopping you from doing things?
- What is it stopping you from doing?
- Can you work through it if you grit your teeth or is it just flat-out stopping you?
- Does it have a name?

If not, let's give it one. This pain is separate from you; it is not you.

- Does it have a color or a shape?
- Does it have feelings?
- How does it make you feel?
- When did it start happening?
- Was it caused by a specific event?
- Or did it gradually show up and now it's really bad?
- Did you wake up with it?

Relieving the Pain

- What are you doing now to relieve the pain?
- Make a list.
- Is it working?
- What works all the time?

- What works some of the time?
- And what doesn't change it?
- Do you have to combine things?
- Is nothing helping?
- What do you think you should be doing for the pain?
- Have other people given you advice about your pain and compared it to their own?

PAST PAIN

Now, let's talk about past injuries that may be contributing to the current situation.

- Have you had foot pain in the past?
- Have you ever experienced this particular situation before?
- Any recollection of this feeling before?
- If so, was it the same or was the pain in the past different from the pain now?
- What did you do before to relieve the pain?
- Did it work?
- Did it work long term?
- Have you had any other injuries in the past?
- What are they?

Make a list; it will help this process.

- Have those past injuries been addressed, or did you just let them heal on their own?
- If you had them treated, what was the process?
- If you "just walked it off," do you remember doing anything yourself to treat it?
- How are those past injuries feeling now?

- Are they gone, still hanging around, or re-irritated now that your foot is hurting?

POSTURE

How is your posture?
- How would you rate your own posture?
- Do you sit for a long time during your average day?
- Do you stand?
- Do you try to do some of both?
- When you notice that you're sitting forward, do you correct it?
- When you're slouching, do you try to correct it?
- Do you know how you got into that position?
- Or how long you have been there?
- What do you do to try to correct your posture?
- Do you "sit up straighter?"
- Do you try to use external tools (such as back or shoulder supports)?
- Have you ever taken a posture class?
- Or watched any posture videos?

Can you relate to looking like a vulture while you're sitting at your desk?

During my knee injury saga, I made some revised body movements that were not great. (Really bad posture, with very little stability.) I didn't even notice them, though, as they were gradually incorporated into my "normal" movements. This happens with your daily posture, as well as when you have an injury. I had lower back and knee injuries rearing their head and some shoulder injuries and a neck injury also contribut-

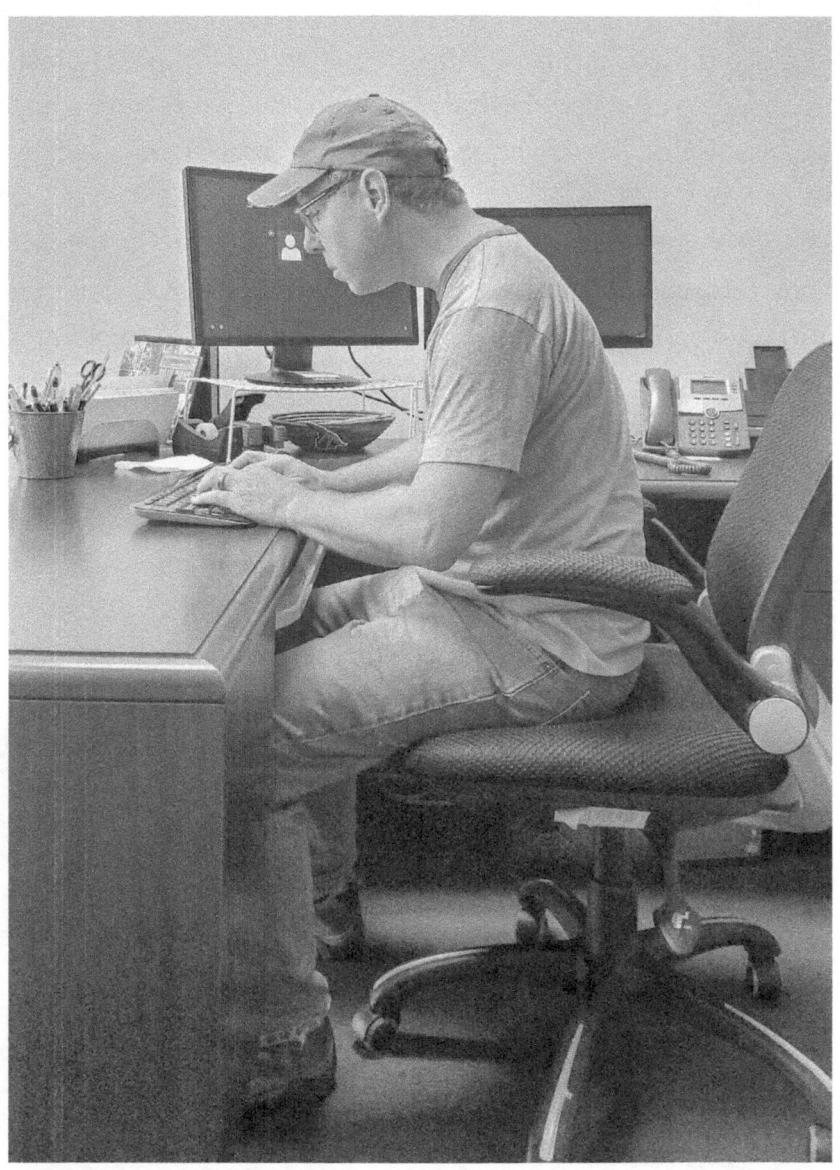

ing. Now, you're asking, "How did all of those other injuries contribute?" As you work through the VITAL ME practice, I will show you. The most important thing to do at this time is to recognize any of your past injuries. Some actually heal and don't contribute—usually if they were treated correctly. Most, however—especially ones that happen when we're young and we just "walk off"—don't necessarily heal or heal the way they started (or we expect).

It's important to recognize that our bodies are doing their best. They compensate for injuries or issues as best as they can at the time. Sometimes these work long term, and sometimes they only work short term, meaning you have to make another compensation down the line. The more short-term compensations you make, the more you make later without even noticing that you're doing it. They are often small things like slightly rotating your foot out, so your knee feels better. That was one of the things I did that led to my foot fracture, and then that same area continued to hurt. I reinjured it unknowingly as my subconscious was trying to protect my knee. I made some other unconscious compensations, too, which we will unravel as we go.

KNOWING WHAT YOUR BODY IS SAYING

At this point, asking yourself all of those initial questions about your pain and really getting to know the pain is really important.

- Pay attention to exactly where it is and where it goes.
- Is it seemingly just in one place, or is it traveling or referring to another place?
- Does anything else hurt?
- What does it really feel like?
- How long has it been there?
- Do you know or is that a mystery too?
- Do you know what started it this time?

Answering the questions of what has happened in the past and how those things were addressed is also important so you can identify if the pain is new, old, or a combination. Take the time to answer the questions as fully as you can. This knowledge is power! This is the most important step in figuring out what is really happening and what will work to get you out of pain.

Sometimes, when a particular place, like your foot, hurts that part is yelling at you so loudly that you don't hear or feel any other part of your body. You need to recognize that pain is a means your body uses to tell you something. You have a painful thing going on and your body is trying to communicate it to you. You will learn to recognize that you are not your pain and that your body is communicating. It's like learning a new language—the body-mind language. When your body tells you something, you will be able to listen and interpret.

It can be challenging when you first start to learn a new language, it seems weird and hard and clunky. Then, all of a sudden, you're in the middle of a conversation and not thinking twice about how to have the conversation or even how you're doing it. This step of really getting to know your pain is crucial. It's laying the foundation for the language. It's like learning vocabulary words.

As you learn to listen and speak to your body and your pain, you will be able to find more creative solutions and sometimes your body tells us the answer.

PAIN AS A CONCEPT

Pain is a difficult concept, as well. You spend the least amount of time as possible in this state. It really takes practice to get to know your pain. You have been taught many things about pain, some by your environment and community, some by your friends and family, and some by your own experiences. Pain is complex. There are many different types, as you have probably experienced. We've heard these described in several ways:

- Pain is bad!
- No pain, no gain!
- If you have pain, take something for it and mask it.
- I can't play anymore if I tell someone something hurts.
- I'll be fine. I'm just going to rest a minute or a few days, months, years.
- It hurts if I do this, so I'll just do this other thing instead.
- It's okay if I cry; someone will attend to me if I do.
- It's not okay to cry; get on with it.
- Rub some dirt on it.

And many more. I'm sure you have several you can come up with on the spot. It's important to remember that these are constructs to help us understand what to do and how to talk to other people about our pain.

Pain is multifaceted and complex, like language. It's not good or bad though; it's your body communicating with you. Some types of pain are more intense than others, so the signal is higher. Your body increased its speaking volume, and maybe sometimes is outright yelling. Learning to pay attention and listen to your body's communication will change the volume that you need to hear it. As you become more adept with your body-mind language you will be able to hear at much lower volumes. When you don't listen or are unaware that you should be listening your body has to get really loud before you pay attention, like this vexing foot pain that has stopped you in your tracks. Your body usually has notified you several times prior to screaming at you that something is not right. You just didn't pay attention or even notice anything was being said to you. You spend lots of time getting your daily tasks done and running here and there, being busy for the sake of being busy, and continuing to add more stuff to your plate. In doing so, you forget to listen to your body. You forget to take care of yourself. You forget to check in, so you check out. If you just keep ignoring a problem, it will go away, right?! You convince yourself of this multiple times a day. Some more evolved people have started to learn some stress control techniques, as you heap more things on your plate all the while. Many of these stress control techniques take you out of your body, your life, and your stress so you can escape for a little while. When you do that, you become less and less able to hear what your body is saying to you, forget how to speak the body-mind language, and have to learn all over again.

If you go back to when you were a young kid, you didn't hide your pain. You told someone right away if you fell, scraped your knee, or your knuckle cracked. Then you got a little older, and some of those made-up pain concepts seeped in, and you changed your behavior around pain and body communication. As you get older and/or busier, you get better at escaping and ignoring. You get worse at listening to your body. Then, you start to blame illness and injury on age or stress instead of doing something about it. If you can relearn how to listen to your body, you can return to better function and less pain.

If you keep going down the pathway of avoidance and disconnection, the problems get more complex and more pain comes with it. You have a tendency to catastrophize your problems and pain, as well. You go from my foot is in pain, to my foot pain is really starting to be a problem, to my foot pain is killing me. It's a fast transition and when you start to catastrophize you can actually make the problem worse because you avoid with more fervor and more of the time. If foot pain is killing you, you will ignore it so it will go away. If foot pain is killing you, then you do everything you can to hide it or cover it up. If foot pain is killing you, you run away from it. If foot pain is killing you, you don't have time for it, so you change your behaviors and your activities. If it's been killing you for a long time, then very often you can't remember what you used to do, how you use to do things, or even what you did to start the issue to begin with because you are so good at avoiding and disconnecting and then telling yourself a story to justify your behavior.

The stories that you make up about your pain can sometimes be a contributing factor to the cause of your pain, as well, or a cause of the behavior alterations you make that then result in compensations and create a negative feedback loop of pain and more compensations—and round and round you go.

EMOTIONS AND PAIN

Emotions can also contribute to pain experiences. Stress can contribute to behavior changes and compensations, too. Emotions contribute to your stories. You sometimes find yourself in positions where your obligations do not allow you to experience an emotional event, positive or negative. When this happens, you have to do something with those emotions, so you usually store them in your body. Very often in your effort to be bigger, faster, stronger in your world, home, and work, you forget to go back and deal with your emotions. So, you continue to store them in your body. Then you add something else when another event happens, and pretty soon you have a layer of emotions that you have made compensations for as well. This creates the same cycle of compensations leading to more pain leading to more compensations. It's like a set of dominos.

Just like in dominos, when you knock the first one down, they all fall down, but unless your dominos were cooler than mine, when you set the first domino back up, the rest don't magically set themselves back up. Sometimes when an initial injury actually heals, all of the compensations you made in the meantime stay present and then cause their own problems and/or pain.

Very often I discuss what emotions have been stored in your body, when we start working with those areas.

Steve was notorious for this. As we were assessing and treating his lower back pain, he would talk about all of the issues he was having with his wife and her family. As we worked through his neck and shoulder pain, he would have something to say about his daughter. Usually, it was something he was worried about or something he knew he couldn't fix for her. Then, as we worked through his foot and calf pain, he would bring up things about his son. He struggled to help his son, who was very sick. As we worked, we discussed that his emotions contributed to his pain. He discovered that he was, in fact, storing all of these various emotions in his body. Together we realigned his body, decreased his pain levels, and reconnected his body to his mind. This allowed him to address his residual emotions. Having an awareness that he was storing emotions was key.

GETTING TO KNOW YOUR PAIN

Getting back to the basics of getting to know your pain and learning how to communicate with your body is important. Identify what your body is trying to tell you. What is it, where is it, what kind is it, and does it go anywhere? Then you can figure out why it is happening, what is actually happening, and how to do something about it. It's important to think about past situations, as well, including stressful situations, emotional situations, a time when you had to keep going, even though you had pain somewhere, a time when you catastrophized the situation, and dive down into behavior changes that you made because of them. Sometimes you make little changes and sometimes you make big changes.

There are many things that may be contributing to your present foot pain: physical pattern or alignment issues, mental issues (pain interpretations), or emotional issues (stressors). Taking the time to learn to communicate with your body is imperative. Your body will tell you what is actually going on if you let it.

Michelle came into my office a complete mess. Everything seemed to be unstable and she was having some nerve issues that were limiting the amount of walking or basic exercise, such as lunges or wall sits, she could do without paying for it for several days after. If she overdid her walking or simple exercise routines she would be stuck in bed or in so much pain she was unable to complete her normal daily routine, even getting dressed. She worked with me to reframe how she classified her pain signals and continues to learn how to listen to her body so she is more aware of when her body is telling her to rest, when it's telling her to limit and stabilize, and when it's okay to push. She has now successfully returned to several of her activities and continues to add more and more exercises and activities.

You can now give yourself a basic assessment. This allows you to listen to your body when it gives you information about what is happening. You can distinguish between various types of pain and what they mean to you and your body. Pain is multifaceted and probably more complex than you thought. You know that your foot pain has many factors contributing to it; it's not just a problem in your foot. And you have some really good reasons to listen to your body.

CHAPTER 5

Improper Alignment—What Is Actually Causing the Pain?

What is body alignment? You will gain a good idea of the answer to this question as you read the next section. There are many parts to alignment. We have the skeletal (bone) and ligament part, the muscles and tendons part, the nerve part, and the emotional part. (I'm talking about stress and disconnection here.) All the parts, or systems, contribute to how your body functions (optimally or not). I'm going to break these systems down, and you're going to get to know how your body alignment compares to optimal alignment and what that means for your movement ability and pain levels.

PATTERNS AND FUNCTION

Now that you have gotten to know your foot pain and some of the things currently and in the past that may be contributing to it, let's talk about how you're functioning and some patterns that you may be experiencing.

If you stood in front of a mirror, what would you see?

- Do you think that you are standing straight?
- Do you think that your shoulders are level?
- That your hips are level?
- Do you think both legs are the same length?
- Both knees are straight?
- Both feet are in the same place?
- Feet pointed the same direction?
- Feet taking the same amount of weight?

Have a look. I'll wait.

What did you see? Take note of it so you can identify some of the patterns that are going on in your body and you can see how they contribute to your foot pain.

- Do both sides of your body feel the same? Probably not.
- Do you have tightness in one calf but not the other?
- Was one knee slightly bent and the other straight?
- One shoulder higher or tighter than the other?
- Was your chin pointing to one side?
- Or your head slightly tilted or rotated to one side?
- Is one hip sticking out farther than the other one?
- Was one foot pointed in one direction and the other in a completely different direction?

I bet that some, if not all, of these things are happening.

- Were you standing up straight in the mirror?

- Or were you questioning your posture ability?
- Can you stand up straight?
- Sit up straight?
- Or do you have to correct and keep correcting?
- Where was your head when you were standing in front of the mirror?
- Rotated, tilted, chin sideways? Which way?

All of these observations will help us figure out what your posture is like and why it has changed over time. This will also help us figure out how these changes have affected your body patterns and function, and how these changes have contributed to your foot pain and any other pain in your body. Again, your pain is your body communicating with you. Let's learn to listen.

Follow this link to download a body diagram: https://body-affects.org/docs/Body-Diagram.pdf. This can help you document what you find.

- What activities do you normally do?
- What is your favorite?
- Are these things compromised by your foot pain?
- What was the motion or thing that officially made you stop completing your exercise?

FOOT-SPECIFIC ANATOMY

Let's get specific about the foot for a minute. The basics of foot anatomy are that it is made up of three groups of bones: tarsals (hindfoot), metatarsals (forefoot), and phalanges (toes). Each part of the foot works independently, but they also all work together. We have patterns between joints, stable-mobile-stable; for example, if the joint in question (like the knee) is stable then the next joint above or below (hip or ankle) is mobile then back to stable for the next one, making a chain. This happens within the foot too. The foot is not one immovable thing. If you hurt a toe, for instance, the toes will become stable (instead of mobile like "normal"). If the toes are stable, then the forefoot becomes mobile (which can lead to pain in between the foot bones, top or bottom, because they are not used to moving). Continuing to follow the pattern, the hindfoot then becomes stable, which can jam the bones that normally move around as you step. This can create pain in the top or bottom of the foot and heel because it's used to moving and now it has to do the forefoot's job. What most people consider to be the ankle is part of the hindfoot; so, the "ankle"/hindfoot becoming stable leads to the knee becoming unstable, and so it continues.

Follow this link for a diagram of the anatomy of the foot. This will help you follow the content more easily. https://body-affects.org/docs/Foot-Anatomy.pdf

As the joints change jobs, so do the muscles, tendons, and ligaments. Tendons become immovable to help stabilize something that is normally mobile, and the ligaments become flexible to allow for movement in a normally stable joint. Everybody wants to play—dominos, here we come.

The foot can affect the rest of the body and the rest of the body can affect the foot; the chain can go either way. Very often, foot pain is not coming from the foot—or not the part of the foot that you think it is.

THE ANATOMICAL BODY

There are a few different ways to look at the body—anatomically (just the muscles and bones, where they are located, and what they're supposed to do), posturally from the top down, posturally from the bottom up, functionally, and optimally functional (optimal biomechanics, which is how the body works at its best, like when you were sixteen and everything worked, nothing hurt, and recovery was lightning fast).

LET'S LOOK AT THE ANATOMY: WAY DOWN TO THE BASICS

When the joints are in alignment, the body movements are a matter of levers. This means when your bones are in the right position and the ligaments are healthy, all the muscles have to do is contract and the movement you want to do happens. For example, bending over to tie your shoe with no restriction or pain.

When the muscles are in alignment, body movements are supported and have more optimal functionality. This means that the muscles are in the right place and healthy, they have no injuries, are connected to the joints via their tendons, and everyone is doing their jobs to make the movement smooth and effortless. For example, picking up a box and placing it on a shelf with no restriction or pain.

There are two main categories of skeletal muscles. The first is mover muscles, which move the bones. The second is postural or stabilizer muscles, which make the movement smooth, stable, and controlled. You need both types to do their jobs or bad things happen. An example of each doing their jobs is walking through a doorway in the middle. Your movements are smooth resulting in your head staying in the middle of your shoulders, each arm swinging the same amount, and your legs moving the same from side to side. An example of when each are not doing their jobs is walking through a doorway and you shoulder-check the side. In this case your head is most likely not in the middle of your shoulders and you are not using your arms and legs the same from side to side because you are using mover muscles to stabilize so they are not able to contract and do their normal movement.

When the nerves are in alignment, the body movements occur at the right time and speed—this means that the other body tissues are receiving the right signal so that the movement you need or want happens when, where, and how you intended at the speed and strength you intended. An example of correct nerve function is picking up a glass of water without crushing or dropping it, without spilling it, and bringing it to your mouth to drink without smashing it into your lip.

Little alterations in these systems happen all the time—your body is not perfect—but you are usually able to correct the issue seamlessly.

It's when big alterations to these systems happen that you begin to have function issues, posture issues, and eventually pain issues. As these alterations get bigger, the body communicates with you. As we have discussed before you ignore these signals. You're really good at it. As you progress through this practice you will learn how not to ignore these little signals. It's much easier to fix a problem when it's little than when it's big and screaming.

POSTURE FROM THE TOP DOWN

This is where your observations come in. Where is your head? The rest of your body follows where your head is, so if it's headed off to the right (pun intended) then so is your body. This means that the muscles on the right side of your body are pulling you over and the ones on the left are trying to figure out how to keep you upright. This is not exactly what their jobs are. They will compensate, though—they're here to help so you can keep going. Off to the left, the opposite happens, tilted or twisted the body follows along. You get the picture. Some of the most common head positions are forward and the body follows suit, usually the upper body moves forward and the lower body is trying desperately to keep you upright. I promise if you lead with your head, you will not get there faster. But you can certainly try. Shoulders also don't make very good earrings, contrary to popular belief, but it happens when you're trying not to let your head get away from you.

POSTURE FROM THE BOTTOM UP

Again, more information from your observations come into play. Where are your feet? The body stacks on top of your feet so if one is going one way, and the other somewhere else, your body gets confused, but it will compensate so you can keep going. If your right foot is pointed out and your left foot is pointed forward, the body follows. The right lower leg follows the foot, then the upper leg follows the lower leg and brings the hip along. Now the whole right side begins to rotate to follow the foot. Meanwhile, the left lower leg stays pointed forward but also has to help keep you upright; then the upper leg tries to help keep you forward and upright, bringing the hip into it. Then, the rest of the left side of the body is stabilizing the lower body and keeping the right side upright. You can see how, if left unchecked, just having one foot rotated a little bit turns into a big problem. Here you have those dominos again, one falls down, so they all fall down (compensation patterns abound). Then, if you set the first one back up (i.e. turn the foot), the rest set up too, right? Not so much. We have to reprogram each part in the series to return to optimal movement.

BODY FUNCTION

When you start to compensate for small things, more and more compensations happen. If you let this pattern run, the posture you would see is a person who has a leg rotated out, likely leaning a little to the right, probably with a high left shoulder (holding him upright), and a head shifting or rotating to the right. These compensations result in a change in function. If you have a foot that is already rotated and you need to rotate it more to walk around something, what do you do? If the foot is already rotated as far as it can go (no movement left), the movement will have to be made from somewhere else. The muscle you would normally use to complete this movement is already being used. This means another joint will have to move or another muscle has to make the movement. This results in that muscle doing the other muscle's job, so now it can't do its own. These movement alterations and muscles doing other muscles' jobs will then continue leading to bigger movement problems or not being able to complete a movement, and eventually pain.

The body really does tell us when little compensations start, you just have to pay attention. One compensation is easier to deal with than the whole set of dominos.

Optimal function occurs when you can seamlessly adjust for the body's imperfections, using your muscles for their own jobs and your joints the way they are meant to move. The goal is to pay attention when your body tells you something is imperfect rather than waiting until it's telling us that something is wrong, or worse yet, screaming at you to stop because it hurts. As you learn to listen to your body-mind language you will be able to stop the issue before it really starts. When we're young kids we are in tune with our bodies—that's why when something happens, like a pop or a scrape, we communicate with ourselves right away. (Did that pop hurt? Is my scrape bleeding?) Then we communicate to others just after that. We're interested in seamlessly correcting the situation so we can continue to play (optimally function).

As you get older and subscribe to outside stresses, emotions, and beliefs, you start to stray away from your body-mind communication. You ignore and allow bigger functional changes to happen before you pay attention or do something. Ignoring your body becomes a pattern and the more you ignore, the worse you get at communicating with your body and the more compensations you make. Your body will compensate and adapt. It's designed to survive. It's also designed to heal. It's pretty good at it. Look at the last time you had a bruise. It was there and then it was gone. Sometimes you ask it to compromise before you allow it to heal. Your body knows where everything belongs and has muscle memory to help it maintain order. If you have asked it to compromise before you allow it to heal, it is no longer in the position where everything belongs, so it may or may not know how to optimally heal. It will heal, but if it doesn't have the guidance it needs, it may heal to a new normal. As you make these new normal healing adaptations, this is where you run into old injuries coming back or contributing to new ones. Your ability to "survive" and keep going is remarkable, but it can also interfere with optimal movement patterns. You make such a small adaptation over a long time that you perceive your "new" normal as normal—similar to my story when I talked about the adaptations I made around my knee when running.

Let's look at what postural adaptations you are starting with. Write them down so as you go through these descriptions you can get an idea of where you're starting.

ADAPTED PATTERNS

Cross Patterns: These happen when one side is not talking to the other. Some muscles are overactive, and some are just not really working. Example: When you walk, you use the opposite arm and opposite leg. If one set of opposing muscles (called a muscle sling, like a cross-body bag) is working well and the other one isn't, you make a compensation. If your right hip is turned out (because of your foot being turned out), the muscles turning your hip out are working overtime and the ones that turn your hip in are not really working. This can cause your left shoulder to be high (to stop you from toppling over to the right) and the muscles elevating your shoulder to work overtime.

Now, let's think about what is happening in the opposite sling—the left hip and right shoulder. If the muscles on the outside of the right hip are working like crazy, the muscles on the outside of the left hip are probably working like crazy, too, not to turn the left leg, but to keep you upright. If the left shoulder is elevated because the muscles are holding you up, what's happening on the right? It's probably not really doing much, or it's pressing down trying to stabilize the rest of the torso. If the right shoulder is pressing down to stabilize, can it do its own job of smoothly moving? No. Then another compensation has to happen so you can keep going.

Stability—Mobility—Stability, Mobility—Stability—Mobility Patterns: When you have your optimal movement patterns intact, you have normal joint function patterns, too. For example, ankles are usually mobile. This allows the foot to be stable on one side and the knee to be stable on the other side. The normal patterns alternate—stable, mobile, stable, et cetera. When these patterns get disrupted with an injury, the patterns shift, but they continue to alternate. In the ankle example, if you sprain your ankle, it becomes stable (usually through swelling or other inflammatory mechanisms). If that is the case than now the foot is mobile and so is the knee. When the chain switches, the joint functions switch and can make you more susceptible to other injuries. So, a normal knee is stable—great. If you injure your ankle, the knee is now mobile—not so good. The knee mobility can lead to ligaments compromising or becoming injured, or muscles being able to pull the knee into positions it doesn't normally go. If you then stabilize the knee before the ankle is ready to be mobile again, you may switch the chain and lead to another ankle injury. Ever wondered why you sprain the same ankle over and over. This is part of that. Also, when the foot is mobile instead of stable, the foot bones can move all over, which can contribute to foot pain. Going back to the idea that the compensations start small, it doesn't take much for your body to accommodate you. If you listen and remediate the issue when it's little, you have a better chance of full healing back to your optimal function. If you wait, the longer you wait and the more compensations that get involved, the more likely you are to create a "new" normal function.

Opposing Joints Pattern: Both sides of your body like to play together, so another way you compensate is from side to side. For example, if your right foot is in pain, then it's likely the left knee will do something funny to help, then the right hip wants to play, too, and so on. Ever feel like your pain jumps? What in the world does your left knee or shoulder have to do with your right foot? This is the answer. Everyone wants to play: your whole body wants to adapt to help you keep going (survive).

POSTURE TYPES

Taking another look at your posture. Let's really break it down to all the sections. Standing posture is different from sitting posture, which is different from lying posture, which is different from all the postures of activities.

It's important to pay attention to what your body tells you, no matter what you're doing. Does your foot pain happen in all of these postures or only some of them? Does one posture help and another one makes it worse? As you break these questions down and observe what the body's telling you, you can learn where the true source of the problem is. Follow the posture. Listen for the muscle tension on one side and not the other, the knee that's not straight compared to the knee that is, the lack of movement in one hip compared to the other, the high shoulder, the tilt of the head.

Is it that stiff neck or wobbly knee that's causing your foot pain? Crazy to think about, right?

Carl came to see me with a sore neck and weird cramps in his hamstrings (the muscles in the back of the thigh). We looked at his body alignment and some of his body movement patterns and found that he was sitting in a forward head posture most of the time. This posture led to his hamstrings overworking to keep him from falling forward. As we worked to correct his alignment and posture through stabilization activities and exercises and some hands-on body techniques, he experienced significant decreases in pain.

Then, after we worked together for a couple of sessions, he found that his neck pain significantly lessened and his hamstrings were getting better, but he developed foot pain. He complained that it was really bad and that he had not experienced this before. We had turned down the pain signals from the other areas of his body, allowing his foot pain to be the loudest. His foot pain was due to his postural alterations and compensations. When his hamstrings were overactive, his calves were also overactive, supporting his body so he wouldn't go too far forward. He demonstrated this posture not only in sitting but also in standing and walking.

The back of his legs and feet were holding on for dear life, trying to stop Carl from toppling forward. The bottoms of his feet were overactive, too. They were contracted all the time, so when he walked around and put his weight through them—not to mention the pull of gravity—those tight muscles resisted the stretch that was being put through them, causing pain. We continued to correct his poor movement patterns and posture and added stabilization exercises to his daily routine. His foot pain, neck pain, and hamstring cramps all resolved. He has successfully maintained his posture, continued his stabilization exercises, and remained pain-free for three years.

By addressing poor movement patterns and postural habits, we were able to eliminate Carl's pain in multiple areas. Recognizing these patterns will help you address your poor movement patterns and in doing so eliminate your pain.

Body alignment is important to function and painful or pain-free movement, wouldn't you say? All the parts or systems of body alignment contribute to the whole and there's more to it than at first glance. How is your alignment and, as a result, how is your body functioning and moving? How do you compare to a pain-free body? Let's find out.

CHAPTER 6

True Patterns—How Do I Understand the Situation?

Now that you have a good idea of what body patterns you have currently, let's have a look at what "normal" pain-free body patterns look like. In this section, you will learn the basics of how your muscles should work and how everything is connected. You'll also learn how movement patterns can be reprogrammed and how your body-mind connection can help (instead of getting in your way).

CORRECT BODY STRUCTURE AND PATTERNS

Understanding body structure, correct and suboptimal, is an important part of really learning how to see and feel your own body's structure. This will allow you to compare your current function to optimal function. As we were discussing, the various patterns that can be present in the last chapter and how they contribute to dysfunction, now you want to look at those patterns and how they contribute to optimal function.

Cross patterning is important for all kinds of tasks; the most common and important is walking. When you walk, you use the opposite arm and leg, and then switch. If you are not doing this, it tells me that there is a problem. When you use, for example, the right leg forward and the left arm forward you are using the muscle sling on that side of the body. When all of the muscles are engaged and doing their job you can walk and run efficiently. In this state, you have the ability to run for long distances. Leiberman and Bramble, leaders in research on human body movement optimization, concluded that we have the capacity to run for longer distances than a horse without risking our health and our lives (see Daniel E. Lieberman and Dennis M. Bramble, "Endurance Running and the Evolution of Homo," *Nature* 432, no. 7015 (2004), 345–52).

In the stable, mobile, stable pattern you have your strongest, most effective joint functions. For example, the hip being mobile allows for the knee to be stable (which, by the way, is how it was designed). Then, the ankle can be mobile and the forefoot stable so the toes can be mobile. If this pattern is occurring, then the hip can swing through its full range for walking, increasing efficiency. The knee then can support the lower leg moving in only one plane (flexion and extension or bent and straightened) not moving side to side, which allows for easy adjustment to uneven terrain at the ankle or the hip. When the ankle is mobile (because the knee is stable), it can adjust for uneven surfaces or direction changes. Then, the forefoot can be stable to support the nerves, muscles, and bones of the rest of the foot. This allows for the tissues (the muscles, tendons, and fascia) to slide and glide smoothly on the sole of the foot (the plantar side), the foot muscles to be supported by the calf muscles, and the nerves between the toes to move freely.

All of these structures can be sources of pain. The fascia, which I like to explain as the mesh between everything else that has a name, encompasses the most pain receptors/detectors. Also, when the forefoot is stable, the toes can be mobile, allowing for the toes to contribute to adjustments to uneven terrain and balance. When this pattern is correct, it allows for balance enhancement as well as the use of what is called ankle and hip strategies to correct your balance. Just as they sound, the ankle strategy is when you use movements at the ankle to regain your balance and the hip strategy is when you use movement at the hip to regain balance. If either one of these joints are not mobile, they cannot move in the ways that you need for regaining balance. If they are "stable" or immovable then it interferes with your walking, running, sitting, and other movements. The same holds true for the upper body and the torso, as the whole-body functions together.

The opposing joints pattern can also be used to optimize the body's ability to use leverage to complete movements more effectively with less effort. If the pattern is correct, then the right hip can move freely, which allows the left knee to effectively stabilize the left leg so when the right foot strikes, the right ankle can move freely into the stride. This pattern means that both sides of the body are working together instead of opposing each other. The same holds true for the upper body and the torso.

There are many more patterns in the body that are subtle; however, if you can understand and optimize these, then the rest come along.

MOVER MUSCLES AND STABILIZER MUSCLES

Now, let's discuss mover muscles and postural/stabilizer muscles. The mover muscles are designed to move the skeletal structure around. The simplest way to look at these is that they turn on during a movement when they are needed and then turn back off when they are not. The simplest way to look at the postural or stabilizer muscles is that they are on a little bit all of the time, monitoring the system, keeping us upright, and stabilizing and supporting the mover muscles when they contract.

If the postural muscles are not turned on, the body is unstable overall. You don't like to be in the state of instability, so your mover muscles often take over for the missing stabilizers. When we are in school and first learning about our bodies, we are taught to run and walk (full body activities), complete sports tasks (whole body activities), and do exercises that strengthen our muscles, such as push-ups and lunges (full body activities). As we complete these tasks when first learning them, our body and brain are working together to create an optimal movement pattern or program. All of our stabilizer or postural muscles are working to stabilize the body as a whole so the mover muscles can figure out how to complete the task. We then move into more focused sports or strength training where we are just concentrating on a single task or single muscles. When this happens at first, we continue to use our stabilizer muscles. As we become less regularly active, because of other obligations like work or family, we start to forget to use our stabilizers. Then, we begin to use our mover muscles to stabilize as well as move, because those are the exercises we remember, and we can make the movement happen regardless of how it looks. I like to say the mover muscles make the movement happen and the stabilizer or postural muscles make the movement happen with grace.

Now, looking back at the basic function of mover muscles, they turn on when you make a movement, then turn back off. If they are being asked to stabilize, then they are being asked to be on all of the time, like a stabilizer muscle, but they are not designed to do that so they fatigue quickly and can be more easily injured, as well. It's important that you are using your correct muscle systems for the correct job and that within those systems, each muscle is doing its own job. Switching up muscular jobs leads to imbalance, some firing too much, some not enough or not at all, and not being able to effectively complete a movement or sometimes not being able to complete the movement at all because there are not muscles available to do the task they are all already busy.

Going back to the basics is hard to do because you can just make the movement happen. You're looking to move with grace. When you do, you are more efficient, effective, and at less risk of injury.

IT'S ALL CONNECTED

Everything in the body is interconnected with everything else. I like to say the nose bone is connected to the toe bone.

This is the domino effect. When everything is optimally aligned and functioning, then it looks graceful and like the domino run right after set-up. The only trouble with this is that it's easy to become unbalanced, and then down go the dominos. If you can stop the process from happening, then you can adjust and correct for the imperfections. If you can recognize the dominos are falling right away, then you can make small adjustments in function before the structure is compromised. If more time passes, more dominos (compensations) fall, the structure begins to be compromised, and down the rabbit hole you go. The sooner you recognize what is happening, the easier it is to correct. This is where it's important to learn to listen to your body, it will communicate the small stuff to you. Your body likes to be able to optimally function.

REPATTERNING MOVEMENT PATTERNS

You can also repattern movement patterns that have been altered. Get your brain to help you instead of being in your way. Some easy examples of this are moving a non-injured body part with an injured one: for example, moving the left shoulder to help the injured right shoulder. You can use the normal or optimal movement pattern of the left shoulder to remind and reprogram the altered movement pattern of the right shoulder back to the same pattern as the left. This works with walking, too. If you find that one foot is doing something different than the other, you can use the optimal movement of the one to help the other.

Another way to help with the reprogramming is to break the short cut programs that you put in your cerebellum (this is the part of the brain you use essentially to automate regularly used movement programs so that you can access them and use them faster and more readily). You break these shortcuts by changing a small movement in the pattern (like changing the angle of your foot when stepping) then you have to go get the original program from the cortex (the optimal movement storage area of your brain) to complete the task.

A great example of this is walking. When you walk forward, you make all kinds of changes to the forward walking program, like accommodating some foot or ankle pain, walking up or down curbs, avoiding other people in crowds, et cetera. The crazy adaptations that you make get stored as a shortcut, so you have them readily available. In order to alter this just enough to need to go get the original optimal program, all you need to do is walk backward for five to six steps. By walking backward, it changes the requirement of walking just enough that the brain has to go get the optimal program for backward walking from the cortex; then when you switch again the short cut has been broken so you have to go get the optimal forward walking program from the cortex. This little reprogram can totally change your gait or walking so that you no longer are hitting a wrong part of your foot, or stop swinging your leg out, or stop limping from that curb check. This is a great example of using your brain to help you instead of getting in your own way.

Normal movement changes all the time and adaptations seamlessly occur most of the time. When enough alterations occur though then the dominos fall. By learning to listen and communicate with your body you can stop things really before they start.

BODY-MIND CONNECTIONS

Understanding the connections between the mind and the body are also important. There have been some schools of thought that indicate that the left brain (the analytical side and the interpreter) is composed of only the left hemisphere of the brain and some connections to the right hemisphere and the right brain (the experiencer and the artsy and emotional side) is composed of both the right hemisphere of the brain and connections and the heart, body, and "spirit." If you follow this line of thinking, then in order to fully experience your world, you have to be in your body, connected to your heart and your spirit, instead of in your head interpreting things. You do not experience your world in your head thinking about things; you experience your world through your senses, all six or more of them (seeing, hearing, smelling, tasting, touching, and intuition or gut sense).

In order to truly function optimally, you have to reconnect and learn to communicate with your body so you can experience everything. Once you experience it, then you can interpret. Your left brain is determined to interpret, and it will even if you have no new information. This is a way you can ignore your body and really disconnect from any pain or emotion that has been stored in your body as well. Unfortunately, much of the meditative world feeds into your desire to escape. It teaches you to disconnect from your body and world by taking your mind up, out, and away. To truly reconnect somatic or body meditation is necessary, this reintegrates your body and mind and helps to open the communication channels between the two hemispheres. You focus your mind on your body and into the structures within (joints, muscles, blood vessels). This is how you learn what you actually feel, what is actually going on, where things are happening, is pain pain, what kind is it, is it anywhere else, is some other part of the body telling you something else, is your body telling you what is wrong, what is not optimal, what pattern you're running or developing. This is really transitioning from learning the vocabulary words to learning how to have a conversation with your body.

OPTIMAL ALIGNMENT

Now knowing what the major patterns of dysfunction are and also how they work optimally, let's break down what is happening with you. Going back to your initial observations and list. Are you functioning optimally? If yes, fantastic! If not, let's see what movement patterns you're actually doing. Standing in front of a mirror will let you see what you are doing, now that you know where and how to look. Where is your head? How about your shoulders? Are your arms the same length on each side? Hip, knees, whole legs? What are your feet doing?

That's a look and comparison of the outside. Let's talk about the inside. How do you feel? Do you know? Are muscles tighter in one area than another? Are your joints feeling the same? Do you feel pretty good but when you look from the outside your shoulders are uneven and your feet are pointed two different directions?

LET'S TRY A SOMATIC OR BODY CONNECTION MEDITATION

I know, it's a scary word—meditation. No, you're not going to be here for an hour—no cushion is necessary, and it's not hard to stay focused. In the beginning, this will be superficial and the more of this you do, the more you will be able to communicate with the deep layers of your body. I find that I can do this with my eyes open or closed at this point in my life, but if you close your eyes, there are fewer distractions from the rest of the world. Your choice.

What I want you to do first is to set a timer for five minutes—yes, five minutes (big time investment here). I'm going to walk you through this and then let you try it. Focus on the top of your head; how does it feel? You don't need to be super in-depth with this. Just note how it feels. Next, move to your neck and shoulders. Note how they feel. Now move on to your arms. Move to your torso. Then draw your attention to your hips and lower back. Next, move to your legs. And finally consider your feet. If you simply note how everything feels, your left brain won't try to make meaning out of it—that's what you want. Just experience. If you take note, your body will tell you what is going on. As I mentioned, this will be just superficial until you practice it. Here are some examples of the type of experiences you may note: slight headache, my right shoulder feels tighter than my left, my hands feel a little numb, my arms feel like they're hanging evenly, I'm able to breathe without pain or effort, my lower back is a little sore, my left hip is throbbing, my left hamstring feels tight, oh, so does my right one, my knees feel locked, my calves feel pretty relaxed, my left foot feels relaxed, my right foot feels like it has a hot poker in the heel, et cetera. Just take note; no one's getting judgy here.

Now turn your timer on and take yourself through your body, head to feet, taking note of what you feel.

- How was it?
- Did you discover anything unexpected?
- Or anything you expected?

The more you go through this little exercise, the better at feeling and listening you will get. You may add a little time, but you should be able to check in and have some idea of how you feel in about five minutes.

As you practice, the sensations you feel and experiences you have will become more detailed. Rather than just noting that your hamstring is tight, you may note that the left outside one is tight and the right inside one is tight. This will help you find what movement patterns are present.

WALKING PATTERNS

Let's look at walking and see if you can recognize how you walk and what happens to your foot when you are walking. Remember, everywhere you go is on your feet, whether you want to or not.

Here is a description of a normal walking pattern. The heel of the foot hits first, then the rest of the heel, rotating just a little toward the outside of the foot, moving through the middle of the foot, crossing over to the area between the big toe and the second toe, and finally moving to the tip of the big toe and leaving the ground. That's just one foot, the other one is doing the same movements on your next step.

- Is that the movement you experience when you're walking?
- Can you pick out any times where something doesn't feel right?

Now, let's talk about some examples of sub-optimal walking patterns.

- Are you turning your foot/feet out too far?
- Or not far enough?
- How about turning in?
- Not hitting your heel first or at all?
- Does your foot feel like a club, like you're stomping from foot to foot?
- Do any of these sound like your steps or, better yet, feel like your steps?

If so, which one? All of these altered movement patterns are your body telling you something. What body movement program happens because of your walking pattern?

Bill had the habit of walking on his toes since childhood. This was an adaptation he made due to a genetic tendon tightness issue. He didn't even know he was doing this or making other adaptations. All he knew was that if he walked for any significant length of time, his feet hurt (like ten minutes). We did an observation activity in front of a mirror so he could recognize this behavior. Then we worked on his tendons, mobilizing and extending them with exercises, stretches, and soft tissue work until he was able to place his heals down and use a heel strike when walking. This changed his stable, mobile, stable pattern in his foot, ankle, and so on. This small change allowed us to address the other posture adaptations he had made and improve his ability to walk efficiently without pain.

As you become more aware of the adaptations that you make, you will recognize what you are doing and be able to use your tools to make relevant changes that will decrease pain and other adaptations.

Here's an example of the stable, mobile, stable pattern. If I'm walking on my toes, then my toes are probably not very mobile, which would then force my forefoot to be more mobile, stabilizing or letting the hindfoot and ankle be less mobile or stuck, making the knee be mobile/unstable, making the hip be stable and immovable.

Here's an example of the opposing joint pattern. If I'm walking on my toes, then my toes are not very mobile. Immobile toes result in increased mobility in the forefoot, which may be painful. The mobile forefoot results in an ankle that is immobile making the opposite knee mobile or unstable. The opposing unstable knee then results in the hip on the same side as the toes being immobile or having to be stable.

Observe how you're walking. Then go back and do your check-in again. See if you can feel what your body is communicating? Can you start to feel the patterns, suboptimal or optimal? How do your patterns compare?

The body is a complex system with many moving parts. However, if you take the time to listen to your body, it will tell you, in a simple way, what you need to know and how to make a change. Making a body-mind connection is crucial. The more you use it, the more you will know what is happening, which will allow you to address your pain quickly and effectively.

CHAPTER 7

Allow for Change—How Do I Manage My Pain and My Expectations?

What do you do with the information your body is giving you? It is important to understand this information, and it can almost feel like a foreign language (which is great if you're good at languages). If you understand the information given to you, a change can be made, optimal movement patterns can be restored, and new ways of interpreting your pain can occur. This information can also inform your healing expectations and help you obtain wins instead of continuing to be frustrated.

WHAT IS PAIN TELLING YOU?

Many people have a skewed notion of what pain is. You think that pain is bad and that you should never have it or that you don't want it. Pain is the body telling you something, just like when your stomach "growls" to tell you that you're hungry. Pain is multifaceted. It can be everything from immediate danger signals—"take your hand off the hot stove"—to "I'm a little uncomfortable or a little ticklish" when someone touches *that* spot. You classify all of those things as painful stimuli in your brain processing system. Pain is also a word you overuse. What I mean by that is that you say something is painful—"I'm in pain. That hurts"—even when you are not experiencing pain. When you tell yourself, your body, your subconscious mind that something is painful, you believe it.

Now, for example, if you were running and experience pain in your foot, that would be an appropriate place to classify that sensation as pain. If you worked out at the gym and were sore the next day, your legs aren't in pain or hurt, per se, but instead are uncomfortable or sore. When you have an in-depth physical therapy treatment or massage you may experience some "pain"; however, if you classify it as productive discomfort, it's placed in a different place in your brain and your experience of it changes. "That hurts so good" is another example of an attempt to reclassify a "painful" stimulus.

It's important that you make these distinctions as they help you to effectively interpret the signals from your body and to alter how you experience these situations. As I said, if everything is "painful," then all of your experiences will be perceived that way. If the body is communicating that something is hurtful to it, like a sprain or a hot stove then you can classify those stimuli as painful and respond appropriately. If you classify a therapy session as productive discomfort (helpful changes being made), you can tolerate more intense or longer treatments, which help the healing process; if, however, you classify those same treatments as "painful," then you can't tolerate as much or as long and the likelihood of the treatment being successful decreases, because your brain has interpreted that something else needs to be done or you have to get away.

This is when you need to rely on the right brain/body to experience what is going on to determine what is actually happening, rather than letting the left brain interpret and classify what is happening. The left brain may or may not have all the information but will make an interpretation anyway. If you give yourself more words, better language to communicate with your body and facilitate the classifications and interpretations of the left brain, you are more likely to heal and heal quickly.

Using words like *pain* or *painful* can be very important. You can also use words like *sore, tender, uncomfortable, unstable, wrong, unhealthy, productive discomfort*, et cetera. You can make your own classifications corresponding to your experience of the stimuli. I look at *sore* and *tender* like I'm working to make myself stronger and faster. Or, I learned a new thing, and my body is getting used to it. I look at *uncomfortable* as something that I need to pay attention to so that I don't move into pain, like it's the first red flag from my body. *Wrong, unhealthy,* and *unstable* are beginning to indicate painful stimuli, like a second red flag. *Productive discomfort* is more like feeling the injury or issue being worked with, noticing that there are beneficial changes occurring in the moment, in the stretch, in the exercise, or in the adjustment, and that the area needs to have close attention paid to it. Not just classifying those sensations in the same category as an initial injury or stimuli that really is a warning can help move through some of the tough work.

Using other words can also help you explain better what is happening to other people, therapists, or yourself. Experiences are very difficult to put into words. Our words don't do justice to what the body is actually experiencing. The saying "a picture is worth a thousand words" is close, but an experience is worth ten thousand words. Your experience of pain in particular can be physical, psychological, emotional, spiritual, or a combination of all of those. You don't really have vocabulary words in language to describe psychological, emotional, and spiritual experiences and are even sometimes lacking in words for physical experiences. Learning to interpret pain in different ways, different words, and different interpretations are important to be able to communicate with your body and to heal.

True healing begins to occur when you stop analyzing your experience and let your body tell you what you need. A great example of this intuitive process is when you bump your knee on the coffee table, your first instinct is to rub it. You don't or can't really "fix" the "pain" by doing this; however, you create a different body experience when you do this. This method of attending to a stimulus is called pain-gate. Pain signals, also referred to as nociceptors, are transmitted to your brain via slow channels, like a side street. Touch signals, like rubbing, are transmitted to your brains via fast channels, like a highway. If you take the highway you get there, wherever there is faster than if you take the side streets. So when you rub your knee after bumping it, the signal from the rubbing (the touch signal) gets to the spinal cord and then the brain faster than the bump (the pain signal), essentially shutting the door to the pain signal, so the brain experiences the situation as touch, rather than pain.

CHANGING THE PAIN SIGNAL AND INTERPRETATIONS

Changing the signal can happen several ways. Pain-gate being one way. Pain-gate occurs by interrupting the pain signal with a touch signal. If you visualize the pain pathway as a side street and the touch pathway as a highway; if you take the highway you get there faster. Therefore, if the pain is taking the side streets, and the touch is taking the highway, touch can get to the spinal cord faster and essentially "shut the door" so you don't interpret/hear the pain. Distraction from pain is another; if you concentrate on something else, you change what the brain is attending to. How you think about pain is another way, if you use some of the alternative classifications we were talking about earlier, like *sore* or *productive discomfort*, your interpretation of the signal is altered to either be more tolerable, a good experience, a reparative experience, or similar, instead of just having pain.

Your interpretation can also affect how treatments work. If you think the medication is going to help, it's much more likely to. If you think the massage is going to hurt or make it worse, then likely that will be the outcome. Your brain is very powerful. Ever heard the phrase, "mind over matter?" This is mind over body. However, you want to use your right brain and body, which is experiential, to be the controller and tell the left, interpreter brain how you want it to classify and how you want it to behave the next time this same stimulus comes up. If you tell it to run the stress-trauma program you will have higher pain levels, more muscular tension, more misalignments, and more negative thoughts associated with the experience. If you tell it to run the healing program, you will have lower pain levels, faster healing, less muscle tension and misalignment, fewer compensations, and positive thoughts associated with the experience.

Which sounds more supportive and helpful? All of the psychological stuff I've read indicates that positive thought, positive reinforcement, positive actions all result in bigger, stronger, faster, better. That sounds better than the stress-trauma program, where stuff hurts more and heals slower.

As you move into changing how you view pain, you can change your expectations of healing. If you think something will heal quickly, then there's a good chance it will. If you think that your tools in your toolbox will be right for the job, chances are they will be. If you have exercises, stretches, activities, and body communication in your toolbox you have a great chance of healing quickly. As you begin to understand what is happening in your body that's resulting in a pain stimulus, what should actually be happening, how to listen to your body and what it's telling you it needs to heal, and setting your mind's classifications and interpretation you set yourself up for success.

Chris was dealing with chronic pain, mostly from past injuries that had not been addressed, which resulted in significant body pain (everywhere). As I reeducated Chris on pain and how we interpret and classify it, he noticed that his "pain" levels were less. This sort of freaked him out at first because he felt better and all we did was have a discussion. He learned how to reclassify and then the true pain areas were addressed and the rest of the "sore spots," as he classified them, responded and usually lessened as we set the rest of the dominos back up. He learned how to use the stabilization activities to reduce his misalignment patterns and functioned in a significantly reduced pain state. Chris is still working on his practice—which is why we call it a practice—and continues to improve his function and decrease his pain.

Reprogramming your interpretation of pain, like Chris, can help you make significant changes to your pain experience.

SETTING YOURSELF UP FOR SUCCESS

Setting yourself up for success also allows you to set goals and expectations that are reasonable and achievable. Getting your mindset about pain and really what you're experiencing in a healing framework is the best way to optimizing body function and healing. Checking in with your body is number one. If you're listening to your body and you follow what is going on, you can identify whether doing work or resting is what your body is requesting. If you're noticing one side of your foot is tight, you'll be able to stretch it. Then, if you notice the other side of your foot is unstable or weak, you'll be able to give it the right exercise or support. As you go through the healing process your body will begin to request different things for the same areas, it's like unwinding a yoyo or pealing an onion.

As you use some of your new tools like checking in and listening to what your body is telling you, you will be able to set little mini goals like checking in daily to see what you need.

When you set mini goals following what the body has communicated then you will have continual victories, leading us down the healing, positive thoughts, positive experience pathway.

There are three legs on the health stool. One is exercise, one is nutrition, and one is rest. Giving your body the support with food and supplements is important so it has those tools to heal. Exercising and stretching have their place to be strong and stable, but rest is really important and most of us forget that one. When you check in with your body, you will find that almost always part of what is being requested is rest in some manner or another. Listening and knowing when to rest or let up will change how you heal and how you view healing.

Resting actually helps us to go back to activities sooner, faster, stronger, better. Part of the body check-in is taking time to rest and communicate with the body.

When you begin to feel better, begin to heal, something I like to call "I feel better" amnesia sets in. When this happens, you have the thought process of "I feel pretty good, I don't need to check in, do those exercises, stretch, drink that much water," et cetera. Setbacks and reinjuries can occur by stopping physical therapy, exercises, or activities too soon. The body can revert back to old patterns or hold part of a new pattern and try to use part of an old pattern at the same time, this may cause a new pain to occur or compensations to happen.

Mark came limping into my office. He had debilitating foot pain. He was diagnosed with plantar fasciitis (again, pain on the bottom of the foot—what a helpful diagnosis). We went through the process of figuring out what was actually happening with his body movement patterns. We then discussed reframing the way he classified pain and how the body is connected. I taught him how to check in with his body, listen to it, and make adjustments as necessary to regain optimal movement patterns and a pain-free foot. He continues to run and continues to use this practice so that when something is suboptimal, he can use his tools and techniques to stop it before it starts. Sometimes he gets too busy and forgets to use his practice and then comes to see me for the fast track. It's good to be needed sometimes.

Just as Mark gets side-tracked with his practice, you will too. That's okay. Just start again.

It's important that you continue to check in with your body. Sometimes it's just those little compensations that start the whole chain again. If you check in and address them when they're little you can seamlessly adjust and continue with that optimal functioning.

MINI-GOALS AND MINI-TASKS

We've all heard the term SMART goals. These are great, but they take a lot of time to lay out and they are very much the left brain running the show. If you use your body check-ins to set mini goals or mini tasks for the day, the exercise, the activity then you can make continual progress with your healing and your positive experience. If you really listen to your body and do what it tells you, you can live in your optimal function most of the time.

I call my program the VITAL ME practice because it is a practice; it will take time to learn to communicate with your body. Your body will continually experience changes with activities, and you will need to go through the practice so that you can make sure that you are listening to what your body needs and are then making those adjustments through reprogramming, stretching, stabilizing, strengthening, and following what your body is asking for. Life is unpredictable so you only have control of yourself and your experiences. If you truly spend time checked into your body, you will be able to live in optimal alignment.

Healing expectations are important because if you have unrealistic expectation disappointment will occur. Managing your expectations allows you to see those mini victories. I know we all want our pain gone yesterday, however, the only way to do that is to pretend it doesn't exist or cover it up temporarily with medication, ice, or heat. If you allow your body to communicate with you, this will allow true healing to occur. This will allow for true experience. If you make small controlled expectations of "I will check in every day" or "I will stretch the area my body told me was tight," you will have success and healing. This will allow you to change the way you experience and classify pain and other uncomfortable experiences.

If you make big expectations, like I will be pain-free in two days or after this one massage or one exercise, then you will be disappointed and not believe that anything will work. I'm guessing that's what's been happening and that's why you are reading this book. There are no silver bullets. It takes some work and willingness to believe to make the magic happen (by magic I mean reduction of pain or relief from it). If you allow yourself small steps and small victories they will add up to be a full bag of tools that you will be able to use no matter what's happening and they will add up to positive experiences that lead to living with less pain.

Pain happens to everyone; some people have more resilience to it than others. This change in how you experience pain, how you view it, how you classify and interpret it, and how you find and address the cause of it will ultimately increase your resilience to it. Learning the body-mind language is key and listening and doing what your body is asking you to do will enhance your ability to function in optimized body patterns.

Practice makes progress, I try to stay away from the word perfection—that one is trouble. The more you practice your practice, the better you will be at identifying what is happening, what should be happening, and what your body needs to reprogram the negative patterns and support the optimal ones. Changing the way that you experience your body and your body in the world, in movement, in exercise, in activity, in stillness will change your ultimate life experience. You have the control and the ability to put all of these tools in practice. The first step is to check in, recognize that you live in your body and embrace it, love it, and take care of it. You only get one. Ever heard the saying, "If I knew I was going to live this long, I would have taken better care of myself?" Well, that's what Steve thought.

Steve came to see me with pain so bad he was ready to stop doing everything, I mean everything. This was a man who had always been active, racing motocross, skiing, snowboarding, hiking, biking, you name it. He was a pretty healthy guy until his pain stopped him. We took some time to discuss what had been happening, what was currently happening, and what had happened in the past so I could see the whole picture of what his body was trying to tell us—well, tell him, but he wasn't listening or didn't know how. We figured out what programs he ran, what he told himself (this is his left brain running the show) about his pain and what it meant and that he was not young anymore and that he shouldn't be doing all of these activities, et cetera. We checked him in with his body.

He learned to communicate with and experience what his body was actually experiencing not listening to the left brain's catastrophic version, which was supported by the doctors and other medical professionals he had seen. He was given his hope back when he actually listened to his body about what was happening. He was running some nonoptimal programs that he adapted and ran for years. He had a major case of the dominos. As we began to peel the onion, he had relief and hope that things in his body could change.

As we reprogrammed his pain classifications and he regularly checked in with his body, even more pain relief occurred, and we were able to tell the left brain how we want him to experience his pain and how he experiences the activities that he does. Long story short, he is now in his late fifties and in the best shape of his life. He's in his optimal function, so much so that he forgets his injury existed or is convinced by his left brain that it wasn't debilitatingly painful. He's as active as ever and skiing and snowboarding longer and better than before; he's bike racing faster than ever, and he's experiencing life through his body (not his brain).

As you become more experienced with your VITAL ME practice, you will be able to experience your world in new ways and function more optimally in it. Be like Steve.

Set yourself up for success; learn how to check in with your body and take the time to understand what it is telling you. (This is one foreign language you want to learn.) Make changes to your pain filing system to inform your healing expectations, help you obtain wins (I mean pain relief), and end the frustration of not knowing what is going on with your foot pain.

CHAPTER 8

Learn Techniques—
What Is the Solution?

T his is the good stuff. Now that you have a pretty good idea of what is going on with your body, your posture, your movement patterns, how they compare with optimal ones, and how disconnected your brain is from your body; let's talk tools, tips, and tricks. In this section are some of the best exercises, stretches, and activities I know to help you stabilize your body, reestablish your optimal posture, and reconnect your body and mind.

THE WORST-CASE SCENARIO

Continuing the discussion of the theory that the left brain (the analyzer) is continually interpreting and making judgments of the information being provided and what it already "knows." It is difficult to change body patterns this way. You think that the safe or self-preserving way to do things is the adapted or compensatory strategies you have developed through previous information and the new information of pain. This part of your brain is only concerned with surviving. Sometimes, in its infinite wisdom, it thinks you have to be hungry, tired, in pain, and self-sabotaging to survive. It thinks in terms of the worst-case scenario, so if all of those things happen then "you will survive." It does not also think in terms of the best-case scenario. This is where the right brain comes in. This is where you experience what is actually happening and where you can reprogram or adapt the program to return it to optimal body function, optimal body alignment. If you do this work on your right brain (which includes your body if you remember), then the information your left brain receives is that best-case scenario, and it starts to interpret the best-case scenario as "survivable" and will integrate that information and use that to determine what is necessary to survive instead of the worst-case scenario.

Let's reprogram in the right brain and change your classification program to "survive the best-case" instead of "the worst-case scenario."

CHECK IN WITH YOUR BODY

One of the first tools I use in the check-in process is the following activity. Try closing your eyes and feeling each part of your body listening to what the body is communicating. If this is difficult, you can try a couple of other techniques first and then come back to this check-in.

A way to decrease the monkey mind—a mind going in one hundred different ways—is the "number one" meditation.

You can complete this meditation for a short period of time or a longer time if you choose. You do not need to do this exercise for a long time for it to be effective. What it does is help reintegrate both sides of the brain (including the right side of the brain that is the heart, the body, and the spirit) calming and slowing the mind down.

Set your alarm for the amount of time you want to dedicate to this. It could be one minute, five minutes, or thirty minutes. Next, you may either do this with your eyes open or closed. I find it easier to do this with my eyes closed for fewer external distractions. Get yourself in a comfortable position, turn your alarm on, close your eyes or open focus (looking at nothing) then think of the number one. You are then going to alter whether it is the number or the word. Spell it out; then you are going to also change the fonts in both letters and numbers, change the color, change the texture, change the pattern, change the size, et cetera. You can be creative here. It does not matter what changes you make or how fast, as long as you are thinking of the number one the whole time. I find when I first start this exercise/meditation I change things pretty fast so I can keep my own attention. Then, as I get into it, I can slow my changes down.

When your alarm goes off, turn it off and take a deep breath. This exercise and meditation can sometimes make you feel a little lightheaded or disconnected for a few minutes, but usually you can just resume your previous activity or go on to the next. By doing this you may then be able to more easily check in with your body.

Another common method I use to connect with my body is a technique where instead of just letting my body communicate with me, I visualize my blood flow. Starting with my feet I think of and visualize the blood moving in and out of my toes and feet, then lower legs, upper legs, torso, arms, hands, neck, head, et cetera. It does not matter what order you complete this exercise/ meditation. Once you have experienced your blood flow it is often easy to do a body check-in reversing the order going from your head to your feet.

As you check in your body will help you decide what parts of your body need to lengthen or stretch and which need to strengthen. As you become more skilled with the check-in your body will tell you which activities to do and sometimes what order to do them in.

LOOK AT YOUR BODY POSITION

After your body check-in, then you move to look at yourself in a reflection or mirror so you can visualize what position your body is presently in. These postures will continually change in response to your inside and outside states. You also have the information you gathered and collected earlier about current and past issues and/or pain, what type of patterns you're running, and where your body posture is currently. All these states continually change, reflecting varying stress, injury, pain, hormone, sleep, nutrition, and hydration states, et cetera. Be kind to yourself and take the time to check in with your body regularly.

If you have a pain spot, your body is telling you what it needs. This is the part of your body you should start analyzing first; do you need to stabilize, strengthen, stretch, or rest?

OPTIMAL BASELINES VERSUS YOUR BASELINES

Where are your head, hips, butt? They are connected to your feet. The body goes where the head goes. Pay attention to what you do or are doing: for example, sitting sideways (throwing yourself in the car), standing chair-shaped (leaning forward), sitting couch-shaped (slumped back), walking with a limp or hip hiked up (especially when stressed or tired), or walking like Quasimodo (dragging a foot or leg behind you). We are master compensators. We will continually adapt to "survive" or at least keep going.

Every part of your body has a core; it's not just your abs. You need to make sure you know how to engage your core for stability, balance, and protection from injury. All of the "core" muscles are postural/support muscles and they work together, so when you engage one, you recruit them all. There are several ways to start this process, which we will cover in this chapter.

HOW TO COMPLETE REPROGRAMMING/CORE ACTIVITIES

It's important to note that when completing body optimization movements or postural reformation activities only 10 to 15 percent of your strength is necessary. However, you may find that when you start practicing these activities, you're using much more than this and can become fatigued. This is okay; as you master these exercises and the postural/support muscles in each of your body parts become stronger, you will begin to unconsciously use the appropriate percentage of muscular contraction for your various activities. Your brain already knows how to optimize these movements and fully support your body, sometimes you just need to remind it what it knows and that you want to use these muscles.

EXERCISES TO REPROGRAM THE BODY

Follow this link for a downloadable copy of these exercises, including pictures: https://bodyaffects.org/docs/Exercises-to-re-program-the-body.pdf. This can help you more easily follow the content.

Head Retraction—In this exercise, you will tuck your chin drawing your head back (make as many double chins as you can). Make sure that you draw your head straight back. Do not raise or lower your chin. This can be completed with or without resistance. (Resistance suggestions: clasped hands behind head, car headrest, or mattress [without pillow].) Complete between three to ten repetitions, holding each for five seconds.

Stretch Scalenes—These are the muscles in the front of the neck. They attach and run in all different directions, so to stretch them you need to use several varied positions. These can be done in any order as long as you complete all six, three on each side. To complete each one, you will need to tuck your hand into your opposite back pocket or tuck it under your leg (sit on your fingers) so that you can keep your shoulder stable (so it doesn't move with you). Next, you will complete the three stretch positions. First, bring your ear toward the shoulder opposite to the side you are stabilizing (hand behind your back or tucking your fingers). This stretch should feel good. You should stretch only until you start to feel a little resistance; it should not hurt, so don't push it. Hold this stretch for three seconds. Second, bring your chin forty-five degrees toward the hand behind your back (or tucked) and look up, moving your head like you're trying to touch the back of your head to your shoulder. Hold this stretch comfortably for three seconds. Third, turn your chin forty-five degrees away from the hand you have behind your back (or tucked) and look up as before, holding comfortably for three seconds.

Head Turning (range of motion increases)—To complete this activity, turn your head as far as you comfortably can to one side, aiming to look over your shoulder. Hold this for three seconds, then repeat, turning your head to the opposite direction and hold again for three seconds. In this activity you should keep your head level, trying not to tilt it in any direction.

Neck Side Glides—To complete this activity, shift your head to the side of your mid-line, keeping your head level (like you're trying to put your ear over the end of your shoulder. Try not to let your head tilt. Hold for three seconds and then repeat on the opposite side.

Neck Circles—To complete this activity, you are going to shift your head to one side (like in the side glide), then shift your head forward (like you're trying to put your chin over your toes), then to the opposite side (like side glides), and then to the back (like a chin tuck). Complete each movement painlessly and try to flow from one position to the next without stopping.

Note: This is not rolling your neck/head. Complete this circle in one direction two to three times then switch directions for another two to three times.

Shoulder Shrugs—Complete this exercise by bringing your shoulders up toward your ears and then slowly lowering them into a gentle stretch (of the trapezius/top of the shoulder muscles). Complete between three to ten repetitions moving slowly and with control throughout each of the repetitions. Start with fewer repetitions and add more as you get more comfortable with the exercise.

Rhomboid and Serratus Anterior Contraction—In this exercise, you will use your muscles to draw the points of your shoulder blades back and down (like they are pointing at the opposite butt cheeks). You can break this down into two movements. One is to bring your shoulder blades together, like you're sticking your chest out. The second is to bring your shoulders down, like in the down phase of shoulder shrugs. Then, complete between three and ten repetitions, holding each one for five seconds. Start with fewer repetitions and increase as you are more comfortable with the exercise.

Note: Taking a deep breath will facilitate a neutral shoulder position after pressing shoulders down or back.

Shoulder Protraction/Retraction—These are like horizontal shoulder shrugs. First, place your arms out in front of you (use a wall to help give you a focus point if it helps you); then press your hands forward, like you are trying to push something away from you. Next draw them back, past your starting point, to complete the opposite movement, like drawing your shoulder blades together (as in the last exercise). Complete between three and ten repetitions, moving slowly and with control throughout each of the repetitions. Start with fewer repetitions and increase as you are more comfortable with the exercise.

External Rotator Strengthening—To help facilitate correct exercise posture, place a folded hand towel under your arm, in your armpit. Then position your shoulder in neutral, at rest like when your arm is at your side, and your elbow at ninety degrees. To complete the exercise, rotate the arm you're exercising out/away from the body as far as possible without turning the body, keeping your forearm level with the floor. This can be completed with or without resistance; such as a weight in your hand or by using an exercise band attached to a wall. Complete ten repetitions and repeat on the opposite side.

Note: Try not to drop the towel. Try to start and stop the motion in neutral, not crossing the body. This exercise should be pain-free, if it is not, decrease the amount of motion (or arc) or resistance or stop.

Pectoral Lengthening (pec major, pec minor, biceps)— To complete this stretch, position your arm at 145 degrees of your arm arc (if you think of having your arm straight out to the side at 90 degrees and having your arm straight up by your ear as 180 degrees, you want about half way between). Next squeeze shoulder blades together (like in the protraction/retraction exercise), then turn your head away from the arm that you are stretching. Hold this stretch for three seconds and repeat on the opposite side.

Note: There is a tendency to drop the arm toward 90 degrees when you turn your head, concentrate on keeping the arm up at 145 degrees.

Stretching the Forearm Flexors—This stretch helps to rebalance the wrists. To complete this stretch, turn one hand so your palm is facing up with your elbow bent, then place the opposite hand around your wrist with your thumb on the underside and grab wrist. Then, pull on the wrist (like you're trying to pull your hand off), extend your hand (stretching your hand, moving the back of your hand toward the back of your arm), and continue the stretch by extending your arm (stretching the inside of your arm). Hold this stretch after you have both positions completed for three seconds. Repeat on the opposite side.

Stretching Finger Flexors—This stretch helps to rebalance the hand muscles. To complete this stretch place palms together making sure your fingertips are also together. Next press one set of fingertips into the opposite (for example, right fingertips press into your left, the right fingers are the "working" ones) and hold the pressure for three to five seconds. Next, relax your hands. Then extend the "working" fingers back (like trying to touch the back of your fingers to the back of your hand), apply some gentle pressure with the "non-working" hand (to create a deeper stretch in the fingers), and hold for three seconds. Repeat with the opposite fingers "working."

Exercising the Diaphragm—The diaphragm is the main muscle you use for breathing. I explain the torso muscles as a barrel to help demonstrate how the muscles are related. The diaphragm is the "lid of the barrel." In order to exercise this muscle, you are going to use thoracic/rib expansion. To complete this exercise, you will first take a deep breath into your belly, then fill up the top part of your lungs, and finally when you feel like your lungs are full sniff (inhaling just a little more air in); then slowly exhale. Complete between three and ten repetitions, breathing slowly and with control throughout each of the repetitions. Start with fewer repetitions and increase them as you get more comfortable with the exercise.

Strengthening the Transverse Abdominis—This muscle is often described as your corset (support). I refer to this muscle at the middle of the "barrel." To complete this exercise, you are going to draw in your stomach (like touching your belly button to your backbone or like you're trying to touch the points of your hip bones together), this is not done using your diaphragm, by holding your breath. If you struggle with this distinction, try to draw your stomach in during an exhale. Complete between three to ten repetitions holding each initially for five seconds and building to ten seconds. Start with fewer repetitions and increase as you are more comfortable with the exercise.

Note: This exercise is easiest when lying down and becomes increasingly harder with sitting and standing.

Strengthening the Pelvic Floor—I refer to this as the bottom of the "barrel." You have two distinct parts to this muscle, the front, which ultimately controls urine flow, and the back, which ultimately controls your anal sphincter. It is best to start by contracting both the front and the back together; as these get stronger, you will be able to contract each part individually. To contract these muscles, you will draw up the pelvic floor (visualize stopping the flow of urine and stopping the passing of wind/gas at the same time), the visualization will allow for the contraction to occur. Begin with five repetitions, holding each for three to five seconds, and build to ten repetitions, holding each for ten seconds. Start with fewer repetitions and increase as you are more comfortable with the exercise. Once you are comfortable with contracting both muscles together and have increased your repetitions to ten, then begin again contracting only the front and then only the back and build up repetitions again.

Sean came in with the thought, "Well, I think I have pain because I'm getting older." He expressed that his body would feel pretty good (strong/stable) and then fall apart out of nowhere; then he would seem to be fine again, but a day or so later, he would "wake up" a mess again. He couldn't seem to put his finger on what was going on, and he was finally tired of going back and forth. So, he sought my help.

As we talked through his activities, both now and in the past, we realized that he went from super active exercising or playing some type of sport nearly every day to only occasionally working out or going for a hike and not playing any of his sports. He started working for a new company that had him traveling all the time, so he drove most of the time and was too tired to do anything in his downtime. He forgot how to use his postural muscles (his "barrel" was not working), so he used his mover muscles for everything. Now, as you know, mover muscles get tired pretty quickly and need to rest. He was asking them to be on all the time, so he was constantly compensating with one muscle or another. No wonder things were fine one minute and painful the next.

As we worked through reeducating his postural muscles through observation and specific activities, exercises, and stretches, he noticed that he had more time feeling good than not. He even incorporated some of his posture activities in the car while he was driving which made him feel better about that. He was able to maintain good posture for longer and longer durations in the car, so he had more energy when he wasn't in the car. He learned to communicate with his body so he could keep each muscle doing their own jobs.

Don't use excuses to put off relearning how to use your postural and stabilization muscles. These will enable you to move with grace again, like when you were sixteen and everything worked, and nothing hurt. None of these activities take up very much time, so that excuse is definitely out.

Pelvic Tilt—To complete this activity, you will tilt your pelvic girdle forward (as if pointing your pubic bone towards the floor), creating an exaggerated arch in your lower back, and then rotate back (pointing your pubic bone toward the ceiling) flattening your lower back. The movement comes from the pelvic girdle, not from leaning forward/backward with your head. Repeat the rock in both directions between two and four times in each direction. Next, you will find the neutral position of your pelvis (you should feel like you are sitting on your sits bones (the bony part of your behind) and your tail bone at the same time).

Note: As your hips return to normal movement, it will become easier to sit and stand in a neutral position.

Side Bending and Quadratus Lumborum Lengthening—This exercise is completed using a wall. You will set up your exercise by leaning against the wall (it helps to place your feet about a foot and a half away from the wall), interlacing your hands behind your head, and then flattening your lower back against the wall, keeping your upper body and head/clasped hands against the wall. To complete the stretch, you will side bend until you feel just the very beginning of a stretch. Then, while keeping the bottom elbow on the wall, peel off the top elbow until you feel a gentle lower back stretch. Hold for three seconds and repeat the other direction.

Hip Stabilization/Orientation—To set up this exercise, you will lie on your back with your knees up and both feet on the floor. You will then bring one leg up to ninety degrees, keeping the other leg in the starting position. To complete the exercise, you will create resistance against the leg bent at ninety degrees by placing both hands against your knee and pressing here (about 10 percent effort/resistance) and at the same time you will press the other foot into the floor (about 10 percent effort/resistance). Hold this resistance in both directions at the same time for five to ten seconds, then repeat on the opposite side.

Gluteal Squeezes—This exercise can be completed sitting or standing, but it is easier in a seated position. To complete this exercise, you will contract/squeeze your gluteal muscles in three stages and release them in three stages. First, contract the gluteus minimus (similar to contracting the back of the pelvic floor); second, contract the gluteus medius (this creates a slight outward pull on the hips, bringing the knees away from each other); and third, contract the gluteus maximus (this is the rest of the cheek). When you release the contractions, release them in the opposite order: max (the majority of the cheek), med (letting knees come back in a little), and min (like releasing the pelvic floor). Repeat the contractions and releases in order (one, two, three, then three, two, one) for between five and ten repetitions. Start with fewer repetitions and add as you become more comfortable with the exercise.

Add a Core Bridge to the Gluteal Exercise—To complete this exercise you will contract your glutes (min, med, max) and then lift your back and butt up into a bridge position, making sure you are level/in a straight line from knees to the neck. To release you will relax the muscles in the reverse order as you come down from your bridge: max, med, min. Compete between three and ten repetitions. Start with fewer repetitions and add as you become more comfortable with the exercise.

Adding Calf Raises to Core Bridge Exercise—To complete this exercise, you will contract your glutes (min, med, max) and then lift your back and butt up into a bridge position, making sure you are level/in a straight line from knees to the neck. Next lift your heels up as far as you are able. To release, you will relax the muscles in the reverse order: flatten feet, come down from the bridge, and release max, med, and min.

Note: This can be done lying, sitting, or standing, with each being progressively harder.

Stretching the Iliopsoas—This stretch is for the main hip flexors. To complete this stretch, you will take a big lunge step backward keeping your heel off the floor (take your normal stride length and add two to three inches, staying on your toes), keep your torso upright (like someone hung your head from the ceiling), make sure both hips are pointed forward, then tuck your pelvis (like you're pointing your tail bone to the floor), hold for three seconds. If you need more of a stretch, you can bend your front leg.

Note: This can be done in standing or kneeling.

Hip Mobilization/Fishing—To set up this exercise, you want to be on a bottom stair or stool, making sure you have a place to hold on (for safety). Next you will balance on one leg, using the free leg to complete the exercise, turning your hip in and swinging your leg through like you're dipping your foot into the water. Then do the reverse, going the other way, turning your hip out and swinging in the opposite direction. Complete ten repetitions and repeat on the opposite leg.

Ryan came in to see me after going around and around with all sorts of medical doctors and foot specialists. The verdict they gave him was that no one knew what was causing his foot pain and that maybe it was just in his head. The recommendation was that he should just take high doses of ibuprofen several times a day. Three different doctors told him to do that.

What?

He and I took a look at some of his previous injuries and looked at his current alignment, both at rest and while walking. We discovered that he was running several compensatory patterns and that these resulted in him using his feet in a strange way. He was walking way on the outside of one foot and on the inside of the other one, neither of which is so good for foot function. His hips were becoming more and more stable, changing the mobile, stable, mobile program in his lower body. We worked through regaining alignment, especially in his feet, lower legs, and hips using some soft tissue techniques, body check-ins, and observation.

He also learned how to implement some of the lower body stabilization activities. He incorporated check-ins with his body especially before he goes skiing or snowboarding, so he knows what activities his body is asking for before the primary activity, and then after. He has now been able to go back to his normal exercises and sports with very little feet issues and he has the tools to use if something comes up. And by the way, he's not taking high doses of ibuprofen. "Yay," says his stomach and liver.

Incorporating the exercises and stretches that your body is asking for before another activity or sport can make a big difference. The VITAL ME practice will help you to do this by incorporating body check-ins, like Ryan uses.

Calf Stretches—There are three different stretches completed in this activity. They are equally important so they should always be completed together. First, stretch the gastrocnemius (the big, double-headed calf muscle), in sitting. Place your leg straight and actively bring your toes toward your nose, hold for three seconds. (If you need more of a stretch, you can use your hand or a strap to create some overpressure.) Second, stretch the soleus (the flat muscle underneath the gastroc), in sitting: bend your knee to at least ninety degrees, then actively bring your toes toward your nose, and hold for three seconds. (If you need more of a stretch you can use your hand or a strap to create some overpressure.) Third, stretch your peroneal muscles (the muscles along the outside of your calf), in sitting: tilt your foot so the sole is facing the other leg (make sure you don't have any weight on this leg and make sure there is no pain) and hold for three seconds.

Note: These stretches should always be completed in a non-weight-bearing state (sitting).

Marc came in after years of dealing with his ankle and Achilles tendon being in pain when he would do any sort of major exertion. He was no longer able to run, and he didn't feel comfortable or stable enough to play volleyball. He was starting to lose hope as the doctors told him that he had a bone spur and was going to need surgery.

We began by looking into his body alignment and past injuries and then moved through techniques to check in with his body. As he checked in regularly, he discovered that his body was telling him that different muscles in his calf were firing at the wrong time or not at all. He also learned some things that were contributing to his leg misalignment coming from his head placement and his hip alignment. As he determined what was going on in his body, he completed the stabilization activities that felt productive for the pain he was experiencing. We got him back into alignment with some adjustment techniques and some retraining of his movement patterns. After that, he was able to stabilize his ankle and foot and stretch some of his calf muscles and strengthen others to the point that his pain dissipated. He regained enough confidence to rejoin his volleyball team and is now running happily. He continues to practice checking in every day and also before he exercises so that he can follow his body's requests (when to work out harder or easier and when to rest).

Using body check-ins can help you know when to push an exercise and when to rest, as Marc now knows.

Foot Alphabet—This exercise will help to strengthen all of the ankle and foot ligaments and tendons. To complete this exercise, you will write the letters of the alphabet in the air using your feet. Complete at least one alphabet with each foot, make sure that you switch between capital and lowercase letters as they create different movements. This exercise can be completed in lying, seated, or standing positions.

As you practice each of these activities, your postural/stabilizer muscles will become stronger and more balanced "as a whole unit," and you will reestablish unconscious control of these muscles during various activities. The stabilizer muscles will result in graceful, controlled, optimal movement patterns.

These activities will help with balance and basic movements you take for granted, like sitting to standing or lying to sitting.

BALANCE ACTIVITIES

Follow this link for a downloadable copy of these activities, including pictures: https://bodyaffects.org/docs/Balance-exercise.pdf. This can help you more easily follow the content.

It is important to assess/reassess your balance regularly, so you know where to start or if you need to return to a previous exercise. Balance changes regularly depending on the amount of sleep, stress, focus, hydration, sugar level, injury, compensations, misalignment, muscle tension or soreness you have.

All of these exercises should be completed in a safe environment. I recommend standing in a doorway so you have an easy handhold should you lose your balance.

- Begin by standing using a small base of support (feet close together).
- Progress this exercise by completing the same activity with your eyes closed. When you take your vision away, it increases the difficulty because you overuse your eyes to know where you are both externally and internally. Closing your eyes challenges you to check in with your body's system of knowing where you are in space, called proprioception.
- A more difficult challenge is called tandem standing. This is where one foot is directly in front of the other with your heel touching the toe of your opposite foot. Evenly distribute your weight between your feet. Then

try it with the other foot in front. One side will be easier than the other, and it's not always the same.

- Progress tandem standing by completing the same activities with eyes closed, remember to complete it with each foot in front.
- The next in difficulty is single leg standing: stand on one foot, keeping the leg you are standing on slightly bent (do not lock your knee). Then switch and try the other side. One side will be easier than the other.
- Progress single leg standing by closing your eyes and completing the single leg stance. Remember to complete on both legs.
- You can make all of the above activities even more challenging by completing them on unstable surfaces such as a mat, a BOSU ball, a balance disk, or sand/rocks, et cetera. It's important to complete these activities in order so that you decrease your risk of injury and can confidently complete each activity before progressing to the next more difficult.

Lying to sitting is an activity you take for granted. It is important to practice this so you can maintain your ability and your optimal ability to complete these motions. This is definitely a case of use it or lose it. Try it—you may surprise yourself. "Woah, that used to be easier," you may say to yourself.

Log rolls are the best way to complete this movement because the postural or stabilization muscles can optimally do their jobs and help you maintain body neutral and avoid initiating compensatory strategies. This is the best way to use the torso "barrel." Roll to one side, then push up into sitting. Practice rolling both directions; one way will be easier than the other, but you want to be able to use both.

SITTING AND STANDING

Going from sitting to standing is also important and you are a champ at finding alternative ways to accomplish this move, especially if you've been sitting for a long time (desk worker, I'm talking to you).

Ways to help your body prepare for standing are bending and straightening your knees a couple of times—I call this pumping for joint oil—then complete the pelvic tilts activity from before (while sitting), rock your hips side to side, and flex and straighten your ankles. It really is pumping for oil. Once you've told your body you're moving, now standing will be much easier and feel better.

Sit-to-Stand Optimal Movement Progression

First, scoot to the edge of the chair, then complete the glute exercise from before (min, med, max), and finally stand up. Be careful: sometimes this results in having a much easier time completing the stand, so you over recruit muscles (ask too many to help). Like when you pick up a light thing you thought was heavy. Use your arms to assist you into standing.

To progress the movement, complete the movement without arm assistance. The stronger your postural/stabilizer muscles get, the easier this will be.

Another progression is to practice putting one leg in front of the other to increase the amount of work it has to do; make sure to switch which leg is forward. This will be more difficult if you are trying to do all the work with your mover muscles and really pretty easy if you're using both systems together (this is optimal body movement). Fun, right?

WALKING ACTIVITIES

Walking is a big part of our lives, so learning to walk is a pivotal point for us. Now you get to relearn how to walk. You want to use those original walking programs; they were optimal patterns, you just need to remind yourself that you want to use those programs instead of the current, crazy, or painful ones you've been using.

One of the easiest ways you can break your current walking patterns and return to the optimal one is to become aware of what you are doing. When you gain awareness, you can then reprogram.

Backward walking is one of the fastest ways to reboot or reprogram the compensatory program (that's the painful or crazy one). This simple task allows you to tap into your original walking programs (both backward and forward) without letting your left brain interpret anything. Just five to six steps backward and you have reset your walking programs. Now depending on how long you have been using the compensatory one, you may have to use this trick several times over time to set in the optimal program. Habits have a way of sticking around because your left brain uses them to make judgments. Stick with reprogramming by walking backward and then the "new" old pattern will become the habit.

Simon came in with body aches in his lower and upper back and crazy foot pain especially when he was running. He would try to run through his pain, but he was beginning to lose that battle. He struggled to get any relief, even when he rested, and pain interrupted his sleep. I helped Simon look at his current body positioning and take into account some past injuries, mostly from when he was a kid, that had weakened one ankle more than the other. We then worked together to realign his body, strengthen his cross-body slings, and reprogram his disrupted stability, mobility pattern allowing him to have stable mobility in his ankle again.

We changed how his feet were actually contacting the ground when he ran. He began to check in with his body and is now able to communicate with his body, especially when he runs, so that he can use some of the walking/running reprogramming techniques, like completing them backward when he starts to run a suboptimal pattern. These techniques allow him to return to optimal body movements, seamlessly making changes while he is running. These techniques will also allow you to make those changes to your walking or running.

ACUTE PAIN RELIEF TECHNIQUES

Some additional activities that you can use to decrease really acute pain include resting, which is important, and mobilizing the fascia. Fascia is the webbing in the body—the stuff that's in between and around everything that has a name. The researchers have now found that the majority of your pain receptor or signalers are located in the fascia (see Bruno Bordon and Emiliano Zanier, "Clinical and Symptomatological Reflection: The Fascial System," *Journal of Multidisciplinary Healthcare* 7 (2014), 401–11; David S. Butler and G. Lorimer Moseley, *Explain Pain*

Supercharged: The Clinician's Manual [Adelaide, Australia: Noigroup Publicatons, 2017]).

If you help this tissue to move around freely, then those receptors have less to complain about.

These fascia movement techniques can work everywhere in the body; for an example, I'm going to use the feet. You can use several different things to help move the fascia around—your own hands, your other foot, tennis balls, rollers, et cetera. Do not use these tools the way you have before. There is a significant amount of fascia close to the surface of your skin, so you don't need to apply much pressure to reach it. The fascia is also very sensitive, so you need to treat it gently. You're asking it to move not forcing it to. Let's mobilize the bottom of the foot together.

Begin by checking in with your foot. Listen to what it is saying, how sensitive is it, which side is louder, top or bottom, left or right, toe side or heel side, et cetera.

Next, decide what tool/hand you're going to use to help. Then, visualize that your foot has three sections: toes and ball, midfoot, and hindfoot/heel. Now, gently begin to massage the toe/ball part forward and backward. If that feels good, you can use a little more pressure, but not too much. Then massage side to side. Now repeat the forward/backward massage on the mid foot, then the side to side on the mid foot. Then repeat those on the hindfoot/heel. Once you have made one pass, go back and do all three sections again. If your body communicates with you that you can use more pressure, go for it. But remember the tissue is sensitive, so keep it gentle. More is not better here. After you have made a second pass with each section, you are going to treat the foot as a whole again. Now you're going to use the same forward/backward technique but go all the way from the toes to the heel and back, and repeat side to side on the whole foot too. Repeat on the other foot. Your body likes symmetry.

The foot fascia is now moveable. This will reduce the pain signals, and you should now start to feel more like this is productive discomfort or, even better, a feel-good sensation.

Another technique is rolling through your foot. I recommend doing the fascia mobilization before you do this activity. For this activity, you are going to visualize that your arch has spine segments or levels. Begin with your toes and roll through your foot stacking each level on top of the next, then reverse and unstack the levels. Repeat on the other foot.

Then, you have to roll the foot and the ankle together. Using your toes as a pivot point or the middle of the top, you're going to roll your ankle/foot first one way then the other. Concentrate on making this movement very slow so you can feel each part of the foot and ankle get some lengthening and maintain control of the rolling movement.

THE BODY AS A WHOLE

It's important to look at the body as a whole unit. You are not just one part. (Yes, you're not just your painful spot, even though it seems like it sometimes.) If you use all of these activities together you can reprogram your body so that all of the parts are moving optimally together instead of running those suboptimal compensatory programs. The more you practice these support activities to use your stabilizer muscles optimally, the better able your mover muscles can complete their jobs optimally too.

These tools, tips, and tricks are some of the best; however, they work best if you check in with your body and use the ones you need when you need them. If you spend the time learning how to communicate with your body, you will be able to optimize these tools. You will be able to eliminate pain—all pain, not just foot pain—reasonably quickly and maintain your relief. You will be able to reprogram your body movement patterns and your posture, stop compensatory patterns from getting out of hand, educate and change your pain classification system, and enhance your ability to seamlessly create changes in the moment and in each movement.

CHAPTER 9

My Best Body— Can My Body Stay This Way?

E verything in the body moves together to create efficient, effective, pain-free movement. You have some knowledge of how your body parts connect already. Now, let's look at how that will help you understand neutral body posture. In this section, you will learn how to create movement from a neutral body posture. You will also learn how to develop your neutral body posture and how to use it, during movements, to create a "new" normal pattern (getting rid of "old" compensatory patterns).

BODY CONNECTIONS

Follow this link to download some pictures of body alignment: https://bodyaffects.org/docs/Body-in-Alignment.pdf.

Pictures help you visualize more easily and will help you follow the content.

It is important to understand the connections in the body. The toes are free moving and sit in front of the knee. The ankle supports the bottom of the leg and the knee sits above it, with the hip above that. When the orientation of the body parts is correct, the patterns of movement are correct. If, for instance, the knee moves in front of the toes, then the pressure in the knee joint increases significantly, and the movement pattern suffers; the chain of stability and mobility shifts as the knee becomes mobile to decrease the pressure in the joint. A good example of this occurrence is during a squat. If the movement is done correctly and mindfully, the knee never goes in front of the toes. If the movement is done incorrectly or sub-optimally, the knee goes in front of the toes. Moving through the rest of the body you can use a pendulum to see if everything is sitting correctly on top of or below everything else.

- The head should be in neutral (in the middle of the shoulders, no rotation or side bending).
- The ears should be positioned over the shoulders (not in front of or behind them).
- The shoulders should be positioned above the hips with no rotation, no side bending, no elevation or depression, no rolling forward or backward.
- The midback should be positioned in the middle of the shoulders, not leaning/side bending either way, with no rotation or forward or backward leaning, and with a slight curve to the back.

- The hips should be directly below the shoulders, with no side bending or hip elevation and no rotation forward, backward, up or down.
- The hip bone should be pointing to the front.
- The kneecap should be pointing to the front directly below the hip and the foot facing forward, with no rotation of the leg in or out, no pulling forward or backward, and no knee bending or hyper-straightening
- The outside of the feet should be parallel to each other (not the inside).
- The arms should be handing down to the same point on the leg/hip, not at different heights, with no shoulder rotation or pulling.
- The elbow should be directly above the wrist, and the wrist should be flat, with no forward or backward contraction.
- The fingers should be straight(-ish) and oriented directly below the wrist.
- The arm should be able to rotate so the palm can face forward, toward the body, and toward the back.

All of this should be pain-free if you are in alignment which allows for optimal movement. The body is a delicate balance, so it is important to make a practice out of these activities from the check-in to the exercises and stretches, to change in how you think about and perceive "painful" stimuli.

Dave was about to go in for surgery on his shoulder when he discovered the VITAL ME practice. He worked with me to regain his optimal alignment through soft tissue work and adjustment techniques. Then he started to regularly practice the stabilization exercises and watched his posture and body patterns change, and now he has been able to stay in the moment and in the movement, which resulted in zero surgeries and stronger, more stable movement with his shoulders and body, including overhead movement. Paying attention to what your body is telling you can make a big difference in your capabilities and can help you stay present in your experiences.

All of the body parts interact with all of the other body parts. The foot's movement affects the knee and hip directly, as well as the opposite shoulder and arm, and the torso and neck secondarily with the pass-through or sling movement. Most activities result in opposing movements (that's right arm, left leg, or left arm, right leg). The knee and hip movements affect those same areas and the foot. The movement of the head affects where the rest of the body goes and moves. If, for instance, you are walking somewhere and leading with your headfirst, the rest of your body will follow. Your neck will move forward, and then your shoulders and torso will, too. Then in order to preserve the movement your lower back will contract, and your hips will rotate forward (resulting in your butt sticking out). Next you will ask your legs to move forward, but they have to pull backward to keep you upright (hamstring cramps here we come). Your calves mirror your upper legs so they will be asked to move forward and have to pull backward at the same time to keep you upright (calf cramps, yay). Then the foot will be adapting to the body by staying on the toes, not putting the heels down (it can't get them down because the body is too far forward), resulting in increased pulling and pressure on the middle foot. Sounds great, right? I promise you will not get there faster if you lead with your head.

Now let's look at what happens when you head is in neutral. Your head is upright, and your ears are over the shoulders, not a bad start. You lead with your chest, which keeps your torso upright and your shoulders down and back, without much work. Your lower back can stay neutral (not tight), and your hips remain neutral, allowing you to use your full hip swing and making your walking more efficient. Your leg muscles work together to propel you forward with nothing having to hold you upright and your heel strikes the ground first. Your heel strike allows you to roll through your foot to your big toe and spring off without creating extra pressure or tension. Nicer, right?

NEUTRAL BODY POSTURE

If you use your body from a state of alignment and from a neutral position, you have the ability to perform optimal movements with the least amount of effort.

Debbie had a major ankle sprain and was having a hard time walking. She discovered the VITAL ME practice after eight to nine months of not getting better. She put the stabilization exercises into her daily routine and noticed a change in her walking. She learned how to relate her neutral posture activities to her walking. She then worked with me to accelerate her alignment progress through hands-on therapies and noticed her movement patterns shifting. She learned how to really check in daily and recognize what her body was telling her it needed. She implemented the stabilization activities that her body asked for and sped up her recovery. She was back to pain-free walking in about two months, after almost nine months of pain, altered walking, and frustration.

Learning to start movements from a neutral body posture, like Debbie, will allow you to move much more efficiently and effectively.

I discovered two easy ways to create a neutral posture. (There are several more that are more involved.) The first is the position of your head. The body really does like to go where the head is. Check in and see where your head is—forward, leaning, or rotated sideways? Look in the mirror, too; this can help. Once you know where you are starting from, you can position your head in neutral, ears over your shoulders, no rotation or side bending. Just holding your head in this position begins to make small shifts/changes in the rest of the body. The other way is to position your hips in a neutral position. This is a little more involved, but it starts the same way. Check in to see where you're starting from—use the mirror to help. Are you sitting up really straight? This means you have your hips bent too far and your head forward. Are you sitting like you would sit on the couch? This means you're slumped backward, your hips are rotated backward, and your head is again forward.

Now that you know where you're starting from, you can adjust. Start by completing the hip rotation activity from before. Rock your hips forward and backward a few times in each direction. When you've pumped for some joint oil, you will find the neutral spot. Neutral is when you are sitting on your butt bones (the ischial tuberosities) and the tip of the sacrum at the same time, like a tripod. This position is usually right where you are the least comfortable, at least for now, because this is the position you spend the least amount of time in. This position allows all of your postural/stabilizer muscles to turn on without you having to think about it or work to do so. This change to neutral allows the rest of the body to shift to neutral as well. I recommend doing your rocking seated; it's a little easier. You can do your rocks standing or lying down, too.

Once you have found neutral while sitting, stand up. If you are in neutral when standing you will feel like you are sitting on your thigh bones, your knees will be soft, and your torso will feel lighter. When you stand in neutral, you can stand equally on both feet for a long time, no shifting from side to side throwing your hips out. When you begin movements from neutral postures, the movements are actually easier because all of your muscles are able to do their own jobs (stabilizers stabilizing and movers moving), no compensatory patterns are necessary, and seamless modifications can be made if an imperfect contraction occurs.

HEAD AND HIP STRATEGIES

Head and hip strategies (small subconscious movements) help you regain neutral body positions when they are lost. This can be due to prolonged sitting, uneven ground, tripping, bumping into something, et cetera. You can use either of them to initiate changes throughout the body, but if you use them together, they are stronger and will help improve your alignment faster. The more you practice getting in neutral postures, the more time you will actually spend in neutral postures. This will result in sometimes going to check in where you are and finding that you are already in a neutral posture. It's cool when that happens.

Ben came to see me for some major foot pain. It prevented him from running and doing yoga and interfered with his travel.

He and I discussed what was going on. We reviewed the current situation and his past injuries and issues. Together, we broke down the situation and formulated a plan to get him back in touch with his body, aware of what contributed to his foot pain (the cause really was an issue with a rotated hip and leg, by the way, not his foot).

As he learned how to communicate with his body with meditation check-ins, he learned which stabilization activities his body needed and when. As he implemented these activities and checked in with his body daily, he relieved most of his foot pain in only a couple of weeks. It took a little longer for the pain to fully resolve, as the patterns he reprogramed had been in place for a long time (years) and he had a little bit of "I feel better" amnesia. He would start to feel better and stop checking in and stop doing his stability activities, and it would result in another flair-up of his foot pain. He would get back to his VITAL ME practice, and the pain would immediately decrease and eventually disappear. He continues to practice his body-mind communication. This practice allowed him to figure out what was causing some of his other pain issues as well. Now he's pretty pain-free most of the time.

Learning to use neutral postures to create optimal movement patterns, like Ben, will enhance your ability to be in your best body.

NEUTRAL POSTURE DEVELOPMENT

Neutral postures will help you get more in tune with your optimal movement patterns. When you allow the body to start from a place of neutrality, the movements occur with optimal leverage positions; the joints are free moving, making it easier for us to move the associated bones; and the nerve inputs are moving through open passages so the signals can get where they're going the first time at the right volume. Your body remembers these neutral positions from development. Have you ever seen a toddler learning to walk? They look drunk. They are swaying from side to side. They get their head in front of their body and fall down. They get their head behind their body and fall down. They are all over the place. What they are doing is training the body to find neutral. When they begin to master that neutral position, they use a wide stance to make sure they have it, and then when they really get it, they're off and we can't keep up. Have you ever tried to chase down an efficiently moving toddler? The toddlers don't have any compensation strategies getting in the way of their optimal movement patterns so they can run or walk fast, efficiently, and for a long time. When you add deviations to those original optimal programs, you become less efficient and slower and have less endurance (and maybe even soreness, discomfort, or pain).

BLOOD FLOW AND NEUTRAL POSTURE

Working in stable neutral postures and patterns will also result in increased blood flow and optimal nerve signals. Your tissues will have the blood flow they need to function optimally and to heal quickly if a suboptimal situation arises. This increased blood flow helps with living in a healthy body and also gives your brain the nutrients it needs as well so you can have been regulation of movement, more of that seamless adaptation can occur and less imperfect movements. These postures and patterns also result in optimal nerve inputs, which allow more efficient and effective muscle contractions. When you have efficient and effective muscle movements the bigger more complex, functional movements are better, more stable, more graceful, and more optimal. It all starts with changing the way that you think and the way that you interact with your body.

"NEW" NORMAL

As you become more practiced at starting your movements in neutral and more practiced with the stabilization activities, your body will begin to use those optimal patterns as the standard, the shortcut, and the means of interpreting/allocating meaning. These activities will become your "new" normal state. Practicing these techniques and checking in regularly will allow you to use your right brain/body to tell the left brain what to think. The more you are in this state of neutrality and listening to your body's communication, the easier you will be able to stay in the moment and in the movement. Staying in the moment will help you to notice what your body is telling you in every moment so that you can make small adjustments in real time. The more you stay in the moment, the easier it will be to stay in the movement so that you can experience optimal movement patterns and recognize that you are using optimal body movement patterns. When you are in the movement, you are body-mind connected so that you can avoid injury and/or stop the movement before major damage can occur. This is when you are fluent with your body's communication language. This allows you to listen to all of the small signals your body is giving you as it experiences the world. This allows you to increase your capabilities, be stronger, more stable, and more efficient.

Steve is a great example of this. As he learned how to use his body again and be present in the moment and in the movement, he continued doing all of his activities, and he is stronger and faster with his downhill bike racing now in his late fifties than he was in his late thirties. You can improve your movement patterns, too.

This practice works to change your body patterns no matter what state you're beginning in, whether you're post-injury, "getting older than you used to be," woke up with something going on, or are feeling pretty good. It's about changing how you view "pain" and being able to listen to and communicate with your body. Once this happens, you're like that toddler: off on your way and no one will be able to keep up with you.

Knowing how to obtain neutral body positions and posture will impact all aspects of your life. These neutral patterns will improve your ability to move; you will be able to sustain good posture, be more efficient when walking and running, and more optimally complete exercise-specific tasks (like holding a yoga pose longer, hitting a backhand harder, or lifting a heavier weight). By continuing to practice operating from these neutral positions, you will continually implement "new" optimal movement patterns, and you will regularly eliminate "old" suboptimal or painful patterns.

CHAPTER 10

Experience Body-Mind Check-Ins—How Do I Stay Connected?

I n this section, you will learn about the different sides of your brain and what they do. We will discuss the thinker, protector left brain, and the experiential, sixth sense right brain. You will learn how they can work together in your favor and how to integrate your brain with your body, by completing simple body check-ins. Knowing how to connect the mind to the body will help your body communicate what it needs and when it needs it. This connection practice will allow you to use the items (skills) in your tool belt to stay pain-free.

RIGHT BRAIN, LEFT BRAIN

Really taking the time to understand the connections between the mind and the body is important to develop long-term changes in your perception of pain and your ability to make changes to your movement patterns to allow you to truly experience life. Looking at the connection between the different sides of the brain can help with understanding how your brain functions and why you think the way that you do.

The left brain truly is the analytical thinker. It helps you put your experiences in context and gives meaning to them. This is the part of the brain that "helps you survive." It saves programs and situations around those programs so that you can remember how to run away from the bear or cross the street without getting hit by a car. It also helps you remember how to throw a ball, fish, or jump a fence. The issue with this side of the brain is that it really cannot distinguish between an actual experience and one that it made up.

For example, Billy was crossing the street. He looked both ways and saw no cars, so he began to cross the street. Halfway across, a bike passed in front of him, and then he finished crossing the street. His brain may remember it that way, or it's possible that his brain will store that experience in a much different manner—he interprets that he was crossing the street and almost got hit by a bike, so he has to be prepared for being hit or almost being hit by a bike every time he crosses the street. After Billy stores this information, he can't actually tell you whether or not he almost got hit by a bike; true or not, that's what was stored.

This happens all the time and sometimes it's good and protective and functional, and sometimes it's destructive and actually gets in the way of new experiences. In one way it's good that Billy's brain anticipates being hit by a bike when crossing the road; he's prepared for that event, and sometimes the risk is real. On the other hand, he has a stress response to crossing the street that may alter how he holds his shoulders (they usually go up to your ears when you're stressed), and it may also prevent him from taking the opportunity to cross a new road, like in another country. These files can be reprogrammed. That reprogramming can happen in a few different ways. Some people do personal growth or a type of reprogramming through counseling or things like hypnotherapy. Some people relearn skills or try to reexperience things to alter the file.

Jennifer came in with some pretty significant knee and hip pain. She had some trouble with her feet but didn't think it was related to her other issues. As we worked through educating her about how the body is connected and how misalignment and suboptimal patterns can create compensatory issues, she understood that everything was connected. She even realized that how she held her head at her desk at work actually made a difference in how her knees felt at the end of the day. She checked in with her body daily, and she gave her inner dialogue my voice. She listens to what her body tells her and asks, "What would Julie tell me to do?" This is really her body communicating to her what she needs, but it helps her to give her body my voice; then, she says, she actually listens instead of going back to being disconnected and ignoring it. Jennifer has used the VITAL ME practice to reexperience activities and reclassify pain; in doing this, she altered how her left brain remembers these activities. You can do this, too, and change how you experience everything.

Another way to reprogram is to integrate the other side of the brain. The right side of the brain is intimately connected to and is part of the body. Some people talk about the body or stomach as having a brain, or a sixth sense; these are the experiences of the "body" part of your right brain. Your right brain does not analyze your experiences; it can save some of them (this is muscle memory or pattern memory), but really it just experiences. This is done by using your senses.

When you smell a scent, you simply experience the scent. If you identify what it is or have a memory connected with it, that's your left-brain creeping in. If you taste something, you just experience the different flavors and types of ingredients with your different taste buds, without applying any meaning; it is just experience. Sight and sound are this way, too. Touch and movement (proprioception, knowing where you are in space) are also experiential. These are the types of experiences that this book is focused on.

When you learn a new task, usually you just experience what it feels like. If you then keep learning more about it, you start to store some of the muscle patterns needed to complete the task. A good example of this is walking. When you were a toddler and learning to walk, you experienced the ability to do it and falling a bunch along the way; then you stored the pattern. You still use that stored pattern to walk now. What you have done to it, though, is sent it to a different part of the brain. You have classified yourself as graceful or clumsy or somewhere in between, giving meaning to walking. You used other programs like misjudging where the curb is or moving to avoid running into another person and they have been stored in the cross-reference with the walking meaning file.

You also have another part of your brain, the cerebellum, and it works somewhere in between the left and right brains, creating shortcuts for movement patterns that you use really regularly like deep breathing and walking. When your brain stores a shortcut, it adapts that shortcut quickly as you think or are told by your left brain that you need to. These adaptations are usually protective. So, let's look at the scenario of misjudging the height of a curb. You took that step and the ground was farther away than you thought, so you hit the ground a little bit harder than you meant to. Now the left brain goes you need to protect yourself from that impact so you should hike your hip up a little bit on that side so that foot can't hit so hard. Now you have started a pattern of suboptimal movement. This change leads to a swap of the normal mobile, stable, mobile pattern down the leg. Instead of the hip being mobile it now becomes stabile, the knee becomes mobile, and the ankle stable. You know how that pattern works against you, but the pattern is changed anyway because you gave meaning to the curb misstep. You make changes to your shortcuts all the time. You do not, however, make changes to the original programs. Now you have to reprogram the shortcut.

By checking in with the body, you know what changes have been made and what you need to do to reprogram or deprogram those changes. By knowing what changed, you can use the appropriate stabilization/postural activities to remind the brain what you want to experience or you can use things like walking backward to break the short cut connection and go back to the original program and start the shortcut process over again. You might as well use your brain to help you instead of letting it get in your way.

Pam was having issues with her feet seeming to rotate out (duck or ballerina feet), and then her right knee would hurt. Then, the pain seemed to jump to her left hip. She couldn't predict what would hurt after her feet would "go out," and nothing seemed related or to make sense; the pain jumped all over the place. As she started paying attention to what her body was telling her, the pain patterns became more predictable; she ran a compensatory program where the stability, mobility pattern changed from side to side. She stored these compensatory programs as shortcuts and kept running them instead of optimal movement patterns. Now, she is able to identify when she runs her suboptimal programs and can manage pretty well by completing her stabilization activities, walking reprogramming exercises, and check-ins. Sometimes she still needs some alignment assistance, so she keeps me around.

You truly experience your world in your body or right brain/ body, not in your left analytical brain. By checking in with your body regularly you spend more time in your optimal movement patterns (not your shortcuts) and experiencing the world (not analyzing it).

CHECK-IN PRACTICE

We've discussed a couple of easy ways to check in with your body already. You can use the number-one way, meditation, by focusing on reconnecting both sides of your brain, which calms your crazy left brain down so you can choose to use the right brain, experiential side, instead of the left brain. You can use the blood flow technique, working through the body one part at a time, feeling the blood flowing in and out of each part. You can also use the breath in a similar way to the blood flow.

Has someone ever told you to breathe into a muscle or "into the pain?" This is sort of what they are trying to get you to do. As you experience each part of your body, instead of feeling for the blood moving, you feel for the breath of air moving through each part. These are good ways to begin regularly checking in. Once you get better at using these techniques regularly, you will be able to move into some other more involved techniques. All of these basic techniques can be used for short durations or long ones.

When I first started to use these techniques, I was easily distracted, and my mind would wander off to figure out what a noise was or what else I had on my to-do list or wherever else. This is normal. You ask your brain to process gigantic amounts of information all the time, and with all of our technology, the information load is exponentially more than it was before we had computers. The technique you use is not really the important part; it's the regular use of one. The more you check in with your body, the more you will know about it and what you're experiencing, and the more you will want to check in.

Barb came to me after a bad car accident and was struggling with body pain just about everywhere. She noticed as time went by that her feet significantly hurt. We spent some time figuring out what affected what and how some of her past unaddressed injuries were rearing their heads. We discovered a pattern that she ran and had been running for a long time of leg turn out. She has a history of dance-related injuries, which led to some chain switching (changes in the stable, mobile, stable chain). The car accident exacerbated that chain issue because she was pressing and holding down the brake pedal.

This set of dominos then led her to make other accommodations, and as a result, she experienced "pain" everywhere. As we peeled the layers of the onion back, she regained some body alignment, especially in her legs and feet, and we changed her thought process about pain. She didn't actually have pain, as in something is wrong, everywhere. She had a few areas that were injured or at risk. But she also had some fatigued muscles from compensating for a suboptimal movement pattern, some soreness from muscles working hard to stabilize things they weren't designed for, and some other sensations that were more protective spasms and/or tension limiting motions. All of these various sensations she interpreted as "pain." Not all of them were warning her that tissues were at risk or injured, so we needed to reprogram how she was interpreting and classifying each sensation. This allowed her to determine the difference between injury pain and other signals of varying discomfort, which were her body telling her about suboptimal movement patterns.

As she changed her thought process, she was able to check in and separate different sensations that allowed us to determine what the body needed addressed first, and she ultimately regained strength and stability. She continues to practice her body communication and is pain-free most of the time.

The more you check in with your body, the more it will tell you the best ways to check in and know what you're experiencing. Sometimes this results in creative methods that are all your own—just ask Barb.

Completing check-ins in all positions you use is a good thing, too. Do your blood flow and breath techniques while you're sitting, standing, lying down, kneeling, or completing your stability activities. Whatever positions you find yourself in daily, check in.

We can discuss some more complex ways to check in now but start with something basic and do it often. Again, the important part here is to check in often.

Here are some examples of more complex ways to check in with the body.

Take one part of your body, such as your foot, and have a discussion with it. Ask it how it feels and wait for an answer. Ask it what it needs and wait for an answer. Scan through it looking for specific sensations, are the parts that are supposed to be tight and stable doing their jobs, such as the ligaments connecting the bones together. Are the parts that are supposed to be loose and mobile doing their jobs, like the toes and tendons? You do not have to know what the parts are called or how they work to go through this specific check-in. You have to be aware of what you are feeling and check in with all of the individual tissues in that part of the body.

Move the foot in all of the ways you can move it and ask all of those same questions in every movement. Is every part doing its job? Are they not? Are they doing each other's jobs? Does one movement feel easier or harder than another? Is the movement smooth or choppy? Is it supposed to be? As I said before, the more you check in with your body, the better you will be at understanding what it is telling you and how it tells you. Remember, the body has a brain, too.

Both sides of your brain and your body working together is a beautiful thing. You experience your world through your body/ right brain. Your thinker-protector left brain helps you to stay safe. Your left brain can also get in your way if you do not use your experiential/sixth sense right brain to guide how your left brain interprets, classifies, and stores information. Using regular body check-ins will help you to keep both sides of your brain and your body working together in your favor. Practicing connecting the mind to the body will help you become fluent in the "new" language of your body; allowing it to communicate what it needs and when it needs it. Learning this language and using it regularly will allow you to use the tools in your tools belt to stay pain-free.

CHAPTER 11

Tool Belt on the Shelf—What Happens If I Do Nothing?

W hat's stopping you from finding your solution? Are you procrastinating, making excuses, and continuing to use temporary solutions for your pain? Is it getting expensive? (Most likely.) The VITAL ME practice is a tool belt to help you on your journey to finding a long-term solution to your foot pain. It's important to note that the tools in the tool belt cannot use themselves. The only way this practice will work for you is if you put it into action.

BAND-AIDS AND EXCUSES

Resolving body pain, and specifically foot pain, so you can get back to normal activities, exercising the way you want to, sports you want to play or try, or traveling without interference is invaluable. This is the goal. Learning about and adapting how you classify and deal with pain can help you figure out the sources of pain and then what to do to address the actual problem instead of just treating a symptom and putting a Band-Aid on the issue.

We are fantastic at making up excuses and stories about why we can't address an issue. One of my favorites is "I don't have time." Let's discuss this little nugget. If you continue to deal with your foot pain or other body pain, then you will end up making concessions for where and when you do things and how you get there and get around. The more concessions you make, the more time it takes for you to actually do something. You will have time planning, pick-ups and drop-offs to arrange, extra time to get where you're going (such as to a seat, down an aisle, from the car to a room, et cetera), and time figuring out when you have time for all the rest of the planning. We don't really think actively about these things, but they add up to a big-time suck.

We make up the story of not having enough time to take care of something only to spend more time doing it another way. If you would take just a few minutes a day to check in with your body and learn to communicate with it and then a few more minutes to do a couple of stabilization activities, you have the ability to resolve your pain and sort out the actual cause of the injury so you know how to handle it if it comes back or you do it again. This will actually save you time and hurt. One of my favorite sayings from my stress management class (way back in college) is taking five minutes to do something now will save you thirty minutes doing it later. (This is the truest with dishes, but it works for pain and injury resolution, too.)

We make up other excuses, too. I'll get to my exercises after I do the dishes, take the kids to school, do the laundry, get home from work, wash the cat, blow my nose, staring off into space. Did I mention washing the cat? You know, anything but paying attention to your body or doing your exercises. When we procrastinate, there is usually another fear getting in the way, something like "if I get rid of my pain, I won't get all the attention I've been getting" or "if I do this thing I will fail." Most of these things you tell yourself are untrue, unprovable, and harmful and get in your way. What's the worst thing that can happen if you resolve your foot pain? You have to tell your neighbor how you did it? You resolve it just so it can come back? Well now you have the tools to deal with it quickly if it does come back. Still trying to figure out the worst thing that will happen? Yeah, that's because you made whatever that is into a story and convinced yourself the story was real.

You can come up with a million excuses how not to resolve your foot pain and why you "can't." You're really good at it. All of these will delay your healing journey and cause more of your dominos to fall down. The more dominos that fall the more things that need attention and the longer it will take to resolve everything. As I mentioned before, sometimes the original injury is long healed but the compensatory movement patterns remain and have a life of their own. If you work to resolve your issues early, you will be back to normal faster.

You often get in your own way and then talk yourself into a "good" reason or justification about why you didn't take care of the problem. You do this with housework, work projects, exercise plans, diets, hobbies. You can convince yourself of anything if you try. Your self-talk is exhausting and sometimes surrendering to it is easier than moving into a new space, learning a new program, or resolving pain. Your brain catastrophizes your problems, so if you give yourself permission to catastrophize, then you will justify the worst-case scenario with your self-talk and your excuses. You will make up a grand story about it with lots of details. You can be both the victim and the hero.

There are many excuses you use: time, money, fear, pain, et cetera. These excuses are the number-one reason why most people don't solve their problems. Empower yourself to communicate with your body.

Knowledge (or lack of it) is another huge excuse you use. If I don't know about something, then I cannot be blamed for anything. Selective understanding of and subscription to an issue happens all the time—that way you have the ability to point a finger at someone else if everything goes wrong. Not understanding how the feet interact with the body can get in your way, too, and allow for continued foot pain. Learning to reconnect your head to your body will allow more seamless changes and will allow for increased function.

Peter put off going to get his foot looked at because he thought that he could just rest it and his primary doctor said to stay off it and to take the cocktail of pain killers, muscle relaxers, and anti-inflammatories. He did at one point try the meds, but all they did was make him feel funny, unstable, and unmotivated. He stopped playing soccer and going to the dance club with his friends, which resulted in him doing less and less. His foot pain was just getting worse.

A friend referred him to me, so he thought he'd try just one more thing. He described me as his last hope. He had seemingly tried "everything" with no success. The doctors just told him to take it easy, gave him more meds, and then referred him to the specialist who sent him back to the first doctor (the medical mill experience). He finally decided that he was going to take charge of the situation and knew there was something else out there. He had been dealing with or not dealing with his foot pain for a few years by this point and had pretty much stopped doing all of the things he liked most, wasn't getting much, if any, exercise, and had gained a significant amount of weight. He was pretty hopeless when I first saw him.

He made countless excuses about why he "couldn't" seek any other ways to resolve his foot pain and decided he "was going to have to live with it." By putting off finding a treatment, he spiraled way down into a hole where he was pretty miserable and made the excuse about it, convincing himself that, as the doctors said, "I just have to rest it so I'll keep doing that even though it's not getting better." We began our work of figuring out the cause and him learning to communicate with his body, and things turned around pretty quickly. He's now back to playing soccer on a men's league and going dancing regularly. He made up a pretty convincing story to keep him miserable for a long time. He's glad he's in a new story now.

Michelle put off getting treatment for her back pain because she was "trying to save money." She bought all the back-support pillows, shoe inserts, and self-massage tools she could find.

Some of those products were pretty pricey. She convinced herself that one of these random products was going to do the trick, and when they didn't, she bought something else. All the while "saving money" by not getting help to resolve her back pain. She spent about four years buying all of these random products (she has quite the collection, by the way).

When she finally stopped telling herself that she was "trying to save money," realizing all of the money she had actually spent on all of these products, she was free to pursue a treatment that resolved her issue. She was referred to me by a coworker who had watched all of these products come and go for years, all the while telling her that she should call me. She finally did and we worked together to figure out what was actually causing her pain and I helped her learn to communicate with her body and learn stability activities so that she can stay pain-free by continually making small, seamless adjustments to her routine.

She's now been pain-free the majority of the past two years and happy with her ability to make the changes her body is telling her to. What do we do for money? She was dealing with her pain to save money—what an excuse that was. It was not a good story, but now she has a different story with a better ending.

Does either of these people sound like you? Drowning in your excuses instead of taking action? Both Michelle and Peter finally made the decision to try the VITAL ME practice, and now they have the tools they need to eliminate their pain. Don't wait for your pain to magically go away; start doing something about it.

DOMINOS

Sometimes you think you're doing okay. You just have the occasional sore spot here or there; probably age right? Those "sore spots" are your body communicating with you. If you ignore them, then your body will make compensations for you. Compensatory strategies build on each other. You stub your toe on Monday, and by Friday you're walking like Quasimodo. Sometimes the dominos fall fast, and you compensate quickly and notice a little bit. Sometimes these compensations happen over years, and you don't notice at all until one day someone asks you why you're limping, and you notice that you actually are. Learning to communicate with your body and how to do stabilization activities can stop the dominos from falling. This means that you don't go down the path of small compensations, leading to large compensations, to altered movement patterns, to pain with movement, to pain screaming at us to stop doing whatever you're doing (like running). This is the backslide you want to prevent.

It's much easier to stop an injury before it happens than after; then you can avoid that little thing called pain. If you ignore your body, then the possibility of this pattern happening is pretty high. You ignore, so you compensate; then you ignore because its uncomfortable, and you compensate some more; then you ignore because it's painful and compensate some more until you can't ignore it anymore because the pain and poor movement patterns have stopped you from doing what you want or have to do. As you make compensatory patterns, you start using muscles for each other's jobs and the joints pull in funny ways.

You also forget how to use some of your muscles, so have to accommodate that, too. This is the part where your body actually becomes unstable and your posture goes to pot. Most of us weren't taught a whole lot about how to use and strengthen our postural muscles way back in gym class; we were just taught how to do sit-ups, push-ups, and lunges. So, you don't even know the tools you need to correct these issues if you happen to listen to your body. Making excuses or ignoring your body only leads to backward progression, not toward a pain-free, optimal movement body.

LET'S CREATE YOUR TOOL BELT TOGETHER

I want you to be able to check in with your body to solve your current pain problem and continue to check in and use the stability activities so that you can be in a happier, stronger, and more active body.

If you wear your tool belt, it's there when you need it, and you can add tools to it anytime. If you put it on the shelf, you won't have it when you need it.

I want to help you create your tool belt and fill it with useful tools so that you can figure out the actual cause of your pain and have the tools to do something about it. I want to teach you how to check in with your body and learn to communicate effectively with it. I want to help you learn the activities to stabilize and optimize your body movement patterns. The VITAL ME practice can help you do this, and if we work together, we can figure out the issue and the solution quickly so you can get back to running, skiing, doing yoga, traveling, and all the other things you want to do.

Stop procrastinating, making excuses, and using Band-Aids for your pain. Let the VITAL ME practice help you find a long-term solution to your foot pain. Put this practice and these tools into action; let them work for you.

CHAPTER 12

The VITAL ME Tool Belt

The VITAL ME practice is seven straightforward steps that will enable you to optimally move your body and keep your brain out of your way and working with you. This method is easy to integrate into your daily routine, as it takes only a few minutes each day to check in and find out what your body needs.

USE YOUR BODY WHEN AND HOW YOU WANT

Having pain in your body anywhere can get in the way of being able to do the things you want to do, when you want to do them. Learning to reframe and reclassify pain and pain types, communicate with your body, and follow what it tells you it needs is the best solution I know to remediate pain.

I developed this practice over years and years of gaining knowledge and experimenting on myself through my own injuries and pain. I would like to help you to find the best way to eliminate your pain in a much shorter journey. I did my best to consolidate my knowledge and to combine many modalities, techniques, and activities to give you the most useful, most beneficial, and quickest to help.

THE VITAL ME PRACTICE

In the VITAL ME practice you learn how to assess yourself, using what is currently going on and what has happened in the past to pick apart the situation and figure out what patterns are contributing to the current issue, what is actually causing the problem, and what your body is telling you to do about it. I call it a practice because it is not a one-and-done system. You will go through the whole process over and over as you live your life and have things happen to your body, whether they are accidental or due to overtraining, overdoing, or over-competing. I have an intimate knowledge of my body. I check in daily (at least once), and I know many stabilization and postural activities. And I use this practice over and over as I do crazy things to my body (or stupid things, sometimes).

This practice allows me to try new things, do things I've done since I was a kid, and be as active as I want to be. I still have times where I have to pick through my pain stimuli, to see if it is actually pain or if I'm experiencing some other variation. I have to listen to what my body is communicating to me; is it something that needs to be stretched, stabilized, or do I need to stop what I'm doing and rest (or get outside help). You will be able to really know where the pain is coming from, because most of the time where the pain is located isn't where the problem actually is or, at least, not where it started. Let's find a solution to the problem and not put a Band-Aid over the symptom.

This is one of Steve's favorite steps. He loves the connection between science and art. He came to me and had been through the medical mill, as I call it. He had been passed around and around, and no one could tell him what was going on, why he was in pain, or why nothing helped. They scared him with suggestions of surgery, injections, burning nerves, or having to "just live with it." He was excited when I explained to him how different parts of his body are connected and how they work together (or against each other, as the case may be). He learned how his body worked as a system, and in so doing, he could wrap his brain around it. Before he learned how things were connected, his body was a mystery, and he was definitely disconnected from it, not knowing what was happening or that anything was wrong until it screamed at him. By gaining some understanding of his body as a system, he understood how checking in is useful and how different activities help "fix" certain parts that then influenced the system.

Your VITAL ME practice takes you through analyzing vexing pain and inappropriate alignments (if you have them). Really getting to know your pain can change your experience of it. It can make the difference between continuing to have your pain and finding a way through it to be pain-free.

Katlin came to me devastated by her pain. She was frustrated and didn't know what was wrong. No one up to this point could help her. She had several different pain sensations all mixed together. She had the actual signal of pain that said, "This is injured, and you can't do that movement" coming from her ankle. She also had some muscle ache in her upper calf on the same side and in the whole calf on the opposite side from taking funny steps and redistributing her weight in a suboptimal way. She had some muscle tension and pulled in both of her feet to allow her to keep walking, even with her injury; that was dull, then sharp, then back again. She interpreted all of these signals as the same thing. Everything was painful and both feet hurt "all the time."

As she learned the differences in each of the signals and what her body was communicating to her, she saw a way out of her painful situation. We worked together to stabilize her ankle with certain exercises, so the strain in her muscle could heal. She learned how to check in with her body, specifically with her ankle, so she would know how it was doing and how much activity it could handle each day. These check-ins helped her to regulate her activity, so she was not causing delayed healing and/or reinjury.

She also learned how to change her walking pattern, first to allow for healing by shortening her steps and maintaining a stable ankle, and then to bring herself back to optimal so that her calves weren't working overtime and her feet weren't hanging on to her so she didn't fall over. By reprogramming her walking pattern, she allowed her ankle to heal and eliminate all of the compensatory patterns that were happening to irritate her calves and feet. (And she was able to keep doing what she needed to do.) As she discovered her different pain signals and what they meant, she broke her issues down into bite-sized pieces that she could work through, instead of being overwhelmed by all of the pain signals as a whole.

Your practice will help you learn the difference between true (optimal) movement patterns and the tenacious patterns you develop when you compensate for pain and inappropriate alignments. You make subtle changes in your movement patterns all the time. It's important that you notice and take action when these subtle changes are taking you away from your true movement patterns, getting in the way of normal movement in a muscle or joint, or creating changes in the surrounding areas of your body. The more you recognize these deviations from optimal movement, the faster you will be able to reprogram and return to optimal movement. Noticing when you're beginning to compensate for something will also help you know which stabilization activities will help the most and when you need to ask for some outside help (and who to ask).

Ryan is a hockey player. He has been playing since he was a kid. He's always been an average player, but he loves the game and continues to play on his college intermural team. He increased his skating speed by learning the difference between his altered pattern and the optimal movement pattern. When he was nine, he injured his hips falling off the jungle gym. He landed with his legs splayed out and sprained both hip joints. Since then, he "always" walked with his feet turned out, not just a little bit, but turned out like a ballet dancer. This altered pattern became his new normal, so much so that he didn't know he was doing it. As we worked together through check-ins and observation, he recognized that his feet were, in fact, turned out. When he skated, his feet remained turned out, and he was not able to push off with very much strength. When we reprogrammed his foot position to face forward, in an optimal movement pattern, he increased his push-off strength significantly, thereby increasing his skating speed. Now he's one of the fastest skaters on his team.

Your practice will teach you to allow for changes to happen and keep your expectations reasonable and safe. It will help you to reprogram and reclassify pain and learn how to listen to what your body is communicating to you. You will learn techniques to help you check in with your body and know what you can expect (at that time), tools to reclassify and identify different pain sensations, and tips on which stabilization and postural activities work best to answer the request your body is making. The techniques in the book are my favorites to remediate most problems and they work quickly to help you create optimal movement patterns. Working through your practice with the help of this book, will allow you to change your pain situation.

You now have a mini reference guide of tools to help you reposition and re-posture your body. You will be able to re-stabilize your postural muscles so your mover muscles can do their jobs. Mover muscles allow the movement to occur, postural/stabilizer muscles allow the movement to occur safely, without pain, and with grace. Learn to move gracefully again; using all of your body the way it was intended and connecting your brain and body so that if it's necessary you can make seamless adjustments to a movement pattern.

When Stephanie came to see me, she had some foot pain, but she was determined to continue playing tennis four days a week. She was convinced that she was just going to have to deal with this pain forever.

As we discussed and worked through what was happening, we discovered that she was creating increased foot tension by having altered posture at work and when she was working out. She often went to play tennis after work. Going from her altered posture at work and asking her feet, already tight, to run around on the tennis court exacerbated her pain. As we worked through her postural reprogramming, adding stabilization techniques and stretching, her foot pain lessened. We also changed her expectations of her feet at the same time, by checking in with her body, and were able to change the timing of her tennis so that she did not play after work when her feet were feeling tight. Instead, she would play a little later or would work through her foot tension first and then play. By communicating with her body, she was able to have more appropriate expectations of her body and what it was asking her to do. (When it wanted to or could play tennis.) It's important that you check in with your body so that you know when your body is able to or wants to complete strenuous activities.

TAKE ACTION

We are really great storytellers and can make up excuses with the best. These stories and excuses often get in our way and stop us from taking action. It's important that you acknowledge that you have some of these programs running in the background and then push past and take action, start the practice, and change your pain. Learn how to check in with your body and make it a regular practice. This way you will not be one of the many people who are disconnected from the neck up, have no idea what is actually happening in their bodies, and are surprised when something goes wrong and their body screams at them.

The more you check in with your body, the more you will know and the more you will want to check in. These check-ins allow you to fully experience your body, your environment, and your life. They will help you function optimally for as long as possible, giving you a higher quality of life. They will also help you live in the moment instead of joining the escape movement. Learning to communicate with your body will allow you to be more mindful and respectful of your body, which will reduce the likelihood of causing an issue, injury, or a reinjury. It will also allow you to quickly remediate an issue should it arise, because you won't ignore it and go down the compensation domino run. (Or at least not ignore it for very long.)

When I run, I always check in with my knees first so that I know how they are feeling before I start. This helps me to gauge how far my body wants to and can run. I am also more aware of what my knees are telling me during my run. If I begin to feel some tension, a pinch, or some pain, I can figure out what pattern I began to alter and make a change without having to stop my run. I also know when my knees have had enough and will walk instead of run, if my body tells me to do so. Checking in and listening to my body has made it possible for me to remain active without my ACL and also with all of my battle scars from living an active lifestyle. (You know what I mean.) These check-ins help me plan my stabilization exercises for the day and the week, too. My body knows what it needs so I listen.

I want to help you really know and experience your body, your pain-free body. I want to empower you with tools and awareness to decrease any pain through changes in your body movement patterns, be body aware, and communicate with your body through your body-mind connection.

You now have the techniques, tools, and tips to know how to operate your body. (Wouldn't it be nice if you received a body owner's manual with purchase?) This practice will truly help you to live in your best body. Working directly with me will make some of these transitions happen more seamlessly, make the process easier and faster, and make you more likely to continue your practice.

Use the seven VITAL ME steps to understand your movement patterns, communicate with your body, change your pain, change your life, and get back to exercising.

Acknowledgments

I have been asked to write a book or told to write a book several times in my life. It was finally time, and it was on my terms. I had such a positive experience with this book-writing process that almost since the beginning I have already been considering what my next book will be about. I'm proud of myself for sticking to it and allowing the book to flow through me. Bigger and better things await.

To all of my clients, thank you for trusting me to guide you back to your optimal bodies. And for putting up with the conversions into my versions of your bodies before they became yours.

Gratitude to Roland, your passing was an amazing part of my becoming the practitioner that I am today. Thank you for working with me every day.

Gratitude to Leroy, your passing was instrumental in my journey to find my inner author and to become her, to finding new ambitions and new inspirations, for getting me out of a program of working hard and all the time, and for helping me find life-work balance again.

A special thank you to Patrick for being there when I needed a man.

A special thank you to Amy for lending me your man.

To my friend Samantha, you're an inspiration to me. You have been an emotional rock for me through this process, always checking in, letting me freak out and celebrate, and encouraging me along. You are and will always be in my practice!

A special thank you to my housemate Jeanne Marie, for always encouraging me and not getting annoyed with me taking up the living room to write.

Thank you to my kitty boys, Phantom and Mr. B, for maintaining supervisory vigilance over me and my workspace, keeping good energy around during my writing process, and for the cuddles and keyboard surfing.

To Dr. Angela and all of the people at the Author Incubator, you made the process of writing a book amazing and positive. I'm not exactly sure how you did it, but you went into my brain, organized my thoughts into a book, showed me how to put it on paper, and are helping me help more people. You guys are magical!

Thank you to David Hancock and the Morgan James Publishing team for helping me bring this book to print.

Thank You!

Thank You so much for reading my book, *Conquer Foot Pain.*

I love each and every one of you who opened this book and committed to reading it from the introduction to the conclusion. You're amazing!

Now it's time to start your VITAL ME practice!

As a thank you, I'd like to offer you a free VITAL ME overview webinar. Please email bodyaffects@gmail.com, use the subject line "VITAL ME webinar," and I will send you a link.

I would love to hear about your VITAL ME practice and journey. Please keep in touch at facebook.com/bodyaffects, share your wins. For more resources and information go to www.bodyaffects.org.

About the Author

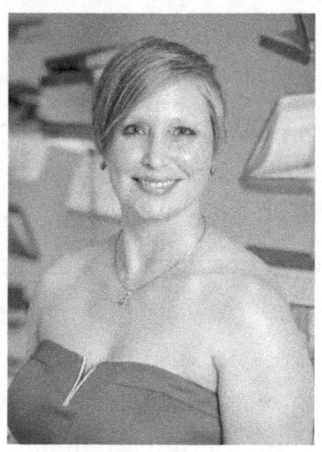

J ulie Smith is the owner and physical therapist of Body Affects. She has been an integrated therapist for over twenty-two years. She is interested in pain mechanisms and reprogramming the body. She specializes in pain relief, helping people work through injuries, pain, and discomfort. She teaches the tools needed to take control of pain or other issues through her hands-on work and her VITAL ME practice.

Julie is a board-certified, licensed physiotherapist—educated in the United Kingdom—a licensed kinesiologist—educated in the United States of America—a nationally- and internationally-certified soft tissue therapist/massage therapist—educated in the U.S.A., U.K., and Thailand—and has pursued continuing education in many fields, leading to additional certifications.

Julie is a native of Colorado, leaving to obtain her education all over the world. She has now been living and working in Colorado for nine years. Her primary practice location is in the Capital Hill area of Denver.

The name of Julie's business represents her practice philosophy. Julie believes that the body affects everything, and we truly experience the world through our bodies.

Julie also has a deep love of elephants and what they represent around the world. Elephants are nature's change-makers, they are family-oriented, they are reverent, and they have amazing memories. Elephants are also thought to bring good fortune, good luck, and to remove obstacles. Julie believes that her life's calling, and her work are all of these things.

Website: http://bodyaffects.org

Email: bodyaffects@gmail.com

Facebook: http://www.facebook.com/BodyAffects

9 781642 798463